**Strategies in Neonatal Care to Promote Optimized Growth and
Development: Focus on Low Birth Weight Infants**

Nestlé Nutrition Institute Workshop Series

Vol. 96

Strategies in Neonatal Care to Promote Optimized Growth and Development: Focus on Low Birth Weight Infants

May 26–28, 2021

Editors

Nicholas D. Embleton Newcastle upon Tyne
Ferdinand Haschke Salzburg
Lars Bode La Jolla, CA

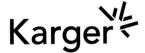

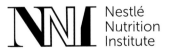

Nestlé Nutrition Institute

© 2022 Nestlé Nutrition Institute, Switzerland
CH-1800 Vevey
S. Karger AG, P.O. Box, CH–4009 Basel (Switzerland) www.karger.com

ISBN 978–3–318–07033–0
e-ISBN 978–3–318–07015–6
ISSN 1664–2147
e-ISSN 1664–2155

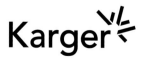

Contents

For more information on related publications, please consult the NNI website: www.nestlenutrition-institute.org

Published online: May 10, 2022

Embleton ND, Haschke F, Bode L (eds): Strategies in Neonatal Care to Promote Optimized Growth and Development: Focus on Low Birth Weight Infants. 96th Nestlé Nutrition Institute Workshop, May 2021. Nestlé Nutr Inst Workshop Ser. Basel, Karger, 2022, vol 96, pp VII–IX (DOI: 10.1159/000519403)

Preface

This book focuses on the challenges of adequately nourishing low birth weight infants in order to facilitate and optimize growth and brain development. These challenges are multiple and require collaboration between clinicians and scientists in order to better understand the underlying mechanisms, and how clinicians can translate this knowledge into clinical practice. The extent and complexity of the data mean that we need collaborative workshops to bring specialties and disciplines together. Whilst the focus of these efforts is relatively easy to define, i.e. low birth weight infants who are born premature, it is more difficult to define the multiple stakeholders. The core stakeholder is of course, the preterm, fragile baby along with their parents and carers who must in turn represent the voice of the baby. Beyond this, there is a need to involve a huge array of health professionals, including pharmacists, dieticians, lactation consultants, nurses, doctors, psychologists, therapists, and many more. Basic scientific support needs to come from experts with detailed knowledge of nutrient intake recommendations, nutrient interactions, gut microbiota, human milk composition such as human milk oligosaccharides (HMOs), growth, body composition, and long-term metabolic and cognitive outcomes. To bring us together requires a huge amount of effort and resource, and there are few forums to do this.

The NNI workshop facilitated interactions between scientists, translation workers and clinicians. The first session "Optimizing Feeding, Nutrition & Growth on the NICU and after Discharge" included discussions how best to start and increase enteral feeds, and next considered the impact of fetal growth and complications such as growth restriction and nutrient requirements. Subsequent sessions discussed the intimate and multifactorial relationship between nutrition and brain growth and went on to consider the continuum of nutritional requirements in the post-discharge period, the challenges associated with the introduction of complementary foods, and how best to meet the challenges associated with eating behaviors. The session concluded with a thought-provoking session on the quality of growth in the NICU and longer-term metabolic outcomes.

The second session "Personalized Nutrition of Preterm Infants" discussed nutritional requirements of newborn preterm infants which depend on birth weight and gestational age. Human milk is the first choice to start feeding, NICUs need to have access to human milk banks to ensure continuous supply but quality of pooled human milk can still be an issue. Protein and amino acid requirements are highest in extremely low birth weight infants (i.e., birth weight <1,000 g), human milk fortifiers provide protein, energy, and micronutrients but their application often interferes with breastfeeding once the infant is mature enough to suckle. Omega-3 (DHA) + omega-6 (ARA) supplementation might contribute to reduce the incidence of severe retinopathy of prematurity, and individualized iron supplementation reduces the risk of behavioral problems. Finally, the promising role of adequate nutrition in modulating long-lasting consequences of early-life stress on brain function and health was addressed.

The third session discussed "The Role of Human Milk Oligosaccharides and the Microbiome in the Health of Very Low Birth Weight Infants." Human milk oligosaccharides (HMOs) are the third most abundant group of components in human milk after lactose and lipids. These complex carbohydrates help shape the developing infant gut microbiome by either serving as prebiotic substrates for beneficial microbes or by directly interacting with host cell biology which can also alters microbial community composition. One specific HMO called disialyllacto-N-tetraose (DSLNT) has been shown in several independent cohort studies to be associated with lower risk for very low birth weight infants to develop necrotizing enterocolitis (NEC). In parallel, infant gut microbial communities are also associated with NEC risk. While data from animal studies corroborate these promising results from cohort association studies, human intervention studies are needed to validate and confirm the beneficial effect of DSLNT in protecting the preterm infant from NEC. Several HMO feeding studies have already been completed in term infants to assess safety and in some cases efficacy, and first HMO feeding studies are now under way in preterm infants as well. While HMOs are currently one of the most studied components, human milk is a complex matrix that contains many more bioactive molecules, microbes, and cells. However, none of these individual human milk bioactives function in isolation. They work in concert and as part of a dynamic biological system that consists of the mother-milk-infant triad, which itself is embedded in a specific environmental context, that can be dramatically different in healthy term infants compared to very low birth weight infants.

The workshop concluded with the notion that it will require a highly functional interdisciplinary team approach and novel, long-term funding strategies to fully understand human milk as part of a biological system with the ultimate goal to improve maternal-infant health and development in general and promote optimized growth and development of low birth weight infants in particular.

Nicholas D. Embleton
Ferdinand Haschke
Lars Bode

Published online: May 10, 2022

Embleton ND, Haschke F, Bode L (eds): Strategies in Neonatal Care to Promote Optimized Growth and Development: Focus on Low Birth Weight Infants. 96th Nestlé Nutrition Institute Workshop, May 2021. Nestlé Nutr Inst Workshop Ser. Basel, Karger, 2022, vol 96, pp X–XI (DOI: 10.1159/000519416)

Foreword

According to the World Health Organization, an estimated 15 million babies are born too early every year. That is more than 1 in 10 babies, and this number is rising.

Early and adequate nutritional support is critical to achieve appropriate rates of weight gain, which are almost twice that of a term infant. Despite intensive nutritional strategies for premature infants, growth failure remains a major problem.

The 96th Nestlé Nutrition Institute workshop took place virtually on 26–28th May 2021. The event was focused on the latest scientific knowledge in the area of neonatal care in preterm and low birth weight infants, including human milk oligosaccharides (HMOs) and their potential impact on the health of neonates.

Speakers discussed the best-in-class nutritional strategies to optimize feeding, nutrition, and growth in preterm infants during their intensive care period and after discharge from the hospital.

The program featured three sessions in which leading international experts provided scientific perspectives on key issues. The first session, chaired by Prof. *Nick Embleton*, looked at optimizing feeding, nutrition, and growth in the neonatal intensive care unit and after discharge. Even with all the efforts to achieve the most appropriate nutrition of preterm babies, intake of key nutrients is still a challenge due to different reasons.

Prof. *Ferdinand Haschke* chaired the second session, which looked at the personalized nutrition of preterm infants. Speakers explained that the contents of breast milk vary over time and are different from mother to mother. Fortification strategies can accordingly be tailored to provide improved support to pre-term infants.

The third session, chaired by *Lars Bode*, looked at the role of HMOs and the microbiome in the health of term and very low birth weight infants. HMOs play an important role in establishing healthy gut bacteria in infants, acting as prebiotics, anti-adhesives/antimicrobials, and epithelial cell modulators. Preclinical evidence shows specific HMOs could help to reduce risk from threats such as NEC in preterm infants. Infant formula with HMOs is safe and well tolerated in term infants as documented in initial studies.

The key issues provided by this 3-day workshop offer valuable insights for healthcare providers, policy makers, and researchers on the crucial role of proper nutrition for adequate growth and consequent development of preterm infants. We gratefully acknowledge the three Chairpersons *Nick Embleton, Ferdinand Haschke*, and *Lars Bode*, who assembled this outstanding scientific program. We would also like to thank all speakers and experts in the audience who have contributed to the content of the workshop and scientific discussions.

Dr. Josephine Yuson-Sunga
Global Head of the Nestlé Nutrition Institute
Vevey, Switzerland

Published online: May 10, 2022

Embleton ND, Haschke F, Bode L (eds): Strategies in Neonatal Care to Promote Optimized Growth and Development: Focus on Low Birth Weight Infants. 96th Nestlé Nutrition Institute Workshop, May 2021. Nestlé Nutr Inst Workshop Ser. Basel, Karger, 2022, vol 96, pp XII–XV (DOI: 10.1159/000519435)

Chairpersons, Speakers and Contributors

Janet E. Berrington
Clinical and Translational Research
Institute
Newcastle University
Newcastle upon Tyne NE2 4HH
UK
j.e.berrington@newcastle.ac.uk

Frank H. Bloomfield
Liggins Institute
University of Auckland
Auckland 1142
New Zealand
f.bloomfield@auckland.ac.nz

Lars Bode
Department of Pediatrics
University of California,
San Diego
9500 Gilman Dr.
La Jolla, CA 82093
USA
lbode@health.ucsd.edu

Ryan S. Carvalho
Nestlé Nutrition
Avenue Nestle 55
CH–1800 Vevey
Switzerland
ryan.carvalho@nestle.com

Kristina Chmelova
Newcastle Hospitals
NHS Foundation Trust
Newcastle University
Royal Victoria Infirmary
Newcastle upon Tyne NE1 4LP
UK
k.chmelova@nhs.net

Carmel T. Collins
SAHMRI Women and Kids
South Australian Health and Medical
Research Institute
Adelaide, SA
Australia
carmel.collins@sahmri.com

Barbara E. Cormack
Liggins Institute
University of Auckland
Auckland 1142
New Zealand
bcormack@adhb.govt.nz

Laura A. Czerkies
Gerber
Nestlé Nutrition
1812 N. Moore Street
Arlington, VA 22209
USA
laura.czerkies@us.nestle.com

Susanne R. De Rooij
Amsterdam UMC
University of Amsterdam
Department of Epidemiology and
Data Science
Amsterdam Public Health Institute
NL–1105 AZ Amsterdam
The Netherlands
s.r.derooij@amsterdamumc.nl

Magnus Domellöf
Department of Clinical Sciences,
Pediatrics
Umeå University
SE–901 85 Umeå
Sweden
magnus.domellof@umu.se

Nicholas D. Embleton
Newcastle Hospitals
NHS Foundation Trust
Newcastle University
Royal Victoria Infirmary
 Newcastle upon Tyne NE1 4LP
UK
nicholas.embleton@ncl.ac.uk

Martijn J.J. Finken
Amsterdam UMC, Vrije Universiteit,
Emma Children's Hospital
Pediatric Endocrinology
NL–1081 HV Amsterdam
The Netherlands
m.finken@amsterdamumc.nl

Kristen L. Finn
Gerber
Nestlé Nutrition
1812 N. Moore Street
Arlington, VA 22209
USA
Kristen.Finn@US.nestle.com

Christoph Fusch
Department of Pediatrics
Nürnberg General Hospital
South Campus
Paracelsus Medical School Nürnberg
Breslauer Str. 201
DE–90241 Nürnberg
Germany
christoph.fusch@klinikum-nuernberg.de

Corinna Gebauer
Human Milk Bank and Division of
Neonatology
Department of Pediatrics
University of Leipzig
Liebigstraße 20a
DE–04103 Leipzig
Germany
corinna.gebauer@medizin.uni-leipzig.
de

Robert A. Gibson
SAHMRI Women and Kids
South Australian Health and Medical
Research Institute
Adelaide, SA
Australia
robert.gibson@adelaide.edu.au

Claire Granger
Newcastle Hospitals
NHS Foundation Trust
Newcastle University
Royal Victoria Infirmary
 Newcastle upon Tyne NE1 4LP
UK
claire.granger@nhs.net

Dominik Grathwohl
Nestle Research Center
CH–1800 Lausanne
Switzerland
dominik.grathwohl@rdls.nestle.com

Nadja Haiden
Department of Clinical Pharmacology
Medical University of Vienna
Währinger Gürtel 18-20
AT–1090 Vienna
Austria
nadja.haiden@meduniwien.ac.at

Ferdinand Haschke
Department of Pediatrics PMU Salzburg
28 Müllner Hauptstrasse
AT–5020 Salzburg
Austria
fhaschk@googlemail.com

Jean-Michel Hascoët
Service de Néonatologie
Maternité Régionale Universitaire
A. Pinard
10 rue du Dr Heydenreich
FR–54035 Nancy
France
jean-michel.hascoet@univ-lorraine.fr

Hannah G. Juncker
Swammerdam Institute for Life Sciences
Center for Neuroscience
University of Amsterdam
NL–1105 AZ Amsterdam
The Netherlands
h.juncker@amsterdamumc.nl

Brian D. Kineman
Gerber
Nestlé Nutrition
1812 N. Moore Street
Arlington, VA 22209
USA
Brian.Kineman@US.nestle.com

Aniko Korosi
Swammerdam Institute for Life Sciences
Center for Neuroscience
University of Amsterdam
NL–1090 GE Amsterdam
The Netherlands
a.korosi@uva.nl

Maria Makrides
SAHMRI Women and Kids
South Australian Health and Medical
Research Institute
Adelaide, SA
Australia
maria.makrides@sahmri.com

Andrew J. McPhee
SAHMRI Women and Kids
South Australian Health and Medical
Research Institute
Level 7, Rieger Building
Women's and Children's Hospital
Adelaide, SA 5006
Australia
andrew.mcphee@sahmri.com

Neena Modi
Imperial College of London
Section of Neonatal Medicine
Faculty of Medicine
Chelsea and Westminster Hospital
Campus
369 Fulham Road
London SW10 9NH
UK
n.modi@imperial.ac.uk

Christopher J. Stewart
Translational and Clinical Research
Institute
Faculty of Medical Sciences
Newcastle University
3rd Floor Leech Building
Newcastle NE2 4HH
UK
Christopher.Stewart@newcastle.ac.uk

Hania Szajewska
Department of Paediatrics
Medical University of Warsaw
Żwirki i Wigury 63A
PL–02-091 Warsaw
Poland
hszajewska@wum.edu.pl

Chris H.P. van den Akker
Pediatrics-Neonatology
IC neonatology (H3)
Emma Children's Hospital - Amsterdam
UMC
Meibergdreef 9
NL–1105 AZ Amsterdam
The Netherlands
c.h.vandenakker@amsterdamumc.nl

Johannes B. van Goudoever
Vrije Universiteit
Department of Pediatrics
Emma Children's Hospital
Amsterdam UMC
University of Amsterdam
Meibergdreef 9
NL–1100 DD Amsterdam
The Netherlands
h.vangoudoever@amsterdamumc.nl

Britt J. Van Keulen
Amsterdam UMC, University of
Amsterdam, Vrije Universiteit
Emma Children's Hospital
Department of Pediatrics
Amsterdam Reproduction &
Development Research Institute
NL–1105 AZ Amsterdam
The Netherlands
b.j.vankeulen@amsterdamumc.nl

Marijn J. Vermeulen
Erasmus MC – Sophia Children's Hospital
Department of Pediatrics – Neonatology
NL–3015 GJ Rotterdam
The Netherlands
m.j.vermeulen@erasmusmc.nl

Published online: May 10, 2022

Embleton ND, Haschke F, Bode L (eds): Strategies in Neonatal Care to Promote Optimized Growth and Development: Focus on Low Birth Weight Infants. 96th Nestlé Nutrition Institute Workshop, May 2021. Nestlé Nutr Inst Workshop Ser. Basel, Karger, 2022, vol 96, pp 1–12 (DOI: 10.1159/000519384)

Starting and Increasing Feeds, Milk Tolerance and Monitoring of Gut Health in Significantly Preterm Infants

Janet E. Berrington

Clinical and Translational Research Institute, Newcastle University, Newcastle upon Tyne, UK

Abstract

Approaches to enteral feeding significantly preterm infants' impact short-term outcomes including survival, late-onset sepsis (LOS), and necrotizing enterocolitis (NEC), and neurodevelopmental and later health outcomes. Clinical practice and trial data are dominated by short-term outcomes (NEC and LOS) with limited longer-term outcomes. Strategies maximizing early maternal breast milk (MOM) exposure and duration of MOM use are key given global health benefits of MOM, but few feeding trials use these as outcomes. Current data support colostrum receipt, early introduction, and progression of volumes between 18 and 30 mL/kg/day, without adverse impact on NEC, LOS, or mortality. Little evidence supports choosing between route of gastric tube placement, bolus, or continuous feed delivery. Individual infants may have specific features that require individualized feed management, such as combinations of growth restriction, antenatal blood flow concerns, intensive supportive needs (including inotropes), and large open patent ductus arteriosus, currently poorly represented in feeding trials. Infant tolerance monitoring includes clinical observations (stooling, abdominal size, vomiting) but routine gastric aspiration appears unhelpful. Infants should be monitored biochemically, anthropometrically, and in the future through bedside microbiomics or metabolomics. Units and networks should audit and compare their rates of mortality, NEC, LOS, neurodevelopment, and growth achieved. © 2022 S. Karger AG, Basel

Goals of Enteral Feeding Significantly Preterm Infants

Enteral nutrition is required for growth and development of a significantly preterm infant (born at <32 weeks' gestation) if they are to be independent of parenteral nutrition (PN) and associated risks and receive maternal breast milk (MOM), with the associated benefits to immune and gastrointestinal (GI) development and function, and reduction in associated risks of necrotizing enterocolitis (NEC), late-onset sepsis (LOS), and neonatal mortality [1]. How and when enteral feeding is established influences these early preterm health complications, and minimizing complications alongside achieving optimal growth and body composition are key goals of preterm neonatal feeding strategies. However, standardizing definitions of NEC and LOS across studies is challenging and agreeing optimal growth trajectories and body composition even more so. Additionally, given the crucial developmental stage of the preterm brain developing ex-utero through the period of what should have been the third trimester, feeding practices directly (via constituents) and indirectly (via the gut-brain axis) [2] impact on neurodevelopmental outcome after early birth. Through metabolic [3] and microbiomic mechanisms, later health outcomes are also influenced [4]. Enteral feeding approaches are therefore a crucial element of neonatal care. Data from infants born <32 weeks' gestation from 13 neonatal intensive care units (NICUs) on 5 continents identified surprisingly large variations in median times to full enteral feeds (range 8–33 days), illustrating wide variations in feeding practices, suggesting cultural as well as scientific influence on feeding practices. Wide variations in clinical outcomes including weight gain achieved (range 5–14.6 g/kg/day), changes in weight z-scores (–0.54 to 1.64), NEC incidence (1–13%) and mortality (1–18%) were shown, but no clear associations between these clinical outcomes and time to full feeds (TFF) [5].

Research Base

Feeding practices in preterm infants are extensively studied: the Cochrane database currently identifies >1,900 trials and 300 reviews on preterm feeding. Interventions are often presented as a simple comparison of one practice against another, but in reality feeding practices are often complex interventions. For example, studies that include an intervention of early milk delivery, or rapid progression will also potentially unwittingly include a decision around whether to wait for sufficient maternal milk (MOM) to implement this strategy, or using an alternative to MOM to allow earlier implementation, and if so, which alternative should be used. Feeding trials are also almost always non-blinded, leading

Table 1. Main evidence base for feeding decisions

Issue	Evidence base		Comment
	clinical outcomes	mechanistic	
Colostrum receipt vs. placebo	Meta-analysis (MA) (2020): NEC ↔ LOS ↔ Mortality ↔	Urinary IgA ↑ Urinary lactoferrin ↑ MOM receipt ↑	MA 9 trials 689 infants [7] Mechanistic studies small [9, 10]
Minimal enteral nutrition vs. none	MA (2013) NEC ↔ LOS ↔ Mortality ↔	None	MA 9 trials 754 infants [12]
Delayed commencement vs. early commencement	MA (2014) NEC ↔ LOS ↔	None	MA 8 trials 1,092 infants [15]
Rate of progression: fast vs. slow	MA (2017) NEC ↔ LOS ↔ Mortality ↔ RCT [18]: PN duration ↓ Motor impairment ↑ Cost ↑	In progress (MAGPIE study)	MA 9 studies 3,576 infants [21]
NG placement vs. OG placement	MA (2013) Time to full feeds ↔	None	MA 2 trials 134 infants [22]
Bolus feeds vs. continuous	MA (2011) Time to full feeds ↔ NEC ↔	None	MA 7 trials 511 infants [24]

to potential bias, and definitions of key outcomes hard to standardize, and not always allied to parental and clinician priorities [6]. Multicenter neonatal feeding trials often leave these options to attending clinicians, allowing recruitment in units with differing approaches, and broad applicability of the results. Single-center studies are often limited to the one approach in use in that unit, making extrapolation of study findings difficult. This chapter focuses on the practical aspects of enteral feeding from birth to the point of established full feeds (TFF) and does not specifically address the issues of what to do if insufficient MOM is available. Table 1 summarizes the key feeding issues, and the current evidence base on which recommendations are made.

Starting Enteral Feeds

Exposure to Buccal Colostrum
Exposure to buccal colostrum sets the scene for receipt of MOM, allowing early exposure of the infant to small volumes of MOM in the first day(s) of lactation without waste. Several small studies have examined the impact of receipt of colostrum, then subject to meta-analysis [7]. Meta-analysis showed no impact on rates of NEC, LOS, or mortality. Individually some of these studies were very small (n = 12–200) and some focused on microbiomic [8] or immunological outcomes [9]. Potentially beneficial changes in urinary lactoferrin, sIgA, and inflammatory responses have been shown [9, 10], but to date without associated demonstrable improvement in short-term clinical measures. Colostrum receipt has been shown to be associated with increased receipt of MOM in infants of median gestational age 28 weeks, at both 6 weeks of age (67 vs. 55%, p = 0.03) and discharge (53 vs. 32%, p = 0.07), in a retrospective case-controlled study after implementation of an oral colostrum protocol [11].

Minimal Enteral Nutrition versus Fasting
Minimal enteral nutrition (MEN) refers to the practice of giving deliberately small volumes enterally for a period of time after birth – also sometimes called trophic feeding. Whether preterm infants should deliberately spend time receiving only MEN before increasing feeds, compared to remaining nil by mouth, has been studied in randomized controlled trials (RCTs) and subject to meta-analysis. Comparison of the incidence of key short-term outcomes discussed above did not identify additional risk from MEN with odds ratios for NEC of 1.07 (95% CI 0.67–1.7), mortality of 0.66 (95% CI 0.41–1.07), and LOS of 1.06 (95% CI 0.72–1.56) [12]. There were 9 trials identified, with the most recent included in the meta-analysis (MA) published in 2008 [13], with 754 included infants. In the included trials, infants deliberately spent at least a week receiving <24 mL/kg/ day after introduction of milk in comparison to a comparable fasting period. The number of infants who were <28 weeks gestation or <1,000 g was small, and the applicability to the most immature of today's infants is uncertain.

Delaying Introduction
The ADEPT study (Abnormal Dopplers Enteral Prescription Trial) [14] explored delaying introduction of first milk until day 6 in comparison to starting on day 2 but did not offer MEN. This group of <35 weeks of gestation infants was high risk by virtue of having both abnormal antenatal Dopplers (absent or reversed end diastolic flow, AREDF) and birth weight <10th centile. Infants who commenced enteral feeds on day 2 achieved full feeds at median age 18 days

(IQR 15–24) in comparison with those waiting until day 6 who were fully fed at median age 21 days (IQR 19–27) with no impact on NEC or LOS demonstrated. This lack of impact on NEC was confirmed in meta-analysis of 8 trials totaling 1,092 infants [15]. There are however data showing clinical benefit of MOM in a dose-dependent manner even in the first 10 days of life, with more MOM positively impacting on survival free of NEC and LOS. This Dutch study took place in a unit without donor human milk using hydrolyzed preterm formula for shortfall in MOM [16]. It has also been shown that the number of days in the first month of life with the proportion of enteral milk that is MOM >50% positively impacts on deep nuclear gray matter volume on MRI (0.15 cm^3/day, 95% CI 0.05–0.25), IQ (0.5 points, 95% CI 0.2–0.8), and motor skills at 7 years of age in infants <30 weeks gestation [17]. Delaying the introduction of enteral feeds with MOM cannot be recommended, but the balance of risks and benefits of feeding strategies in the absence of MOM may differ.

Increasing Enteral Feeds

Rates of Progression
Once first milk has been tolerated, the next clinical challenge is how quickly to attempt to advance milk. Given current understanding of etiology/mechanisms of LOS and NEC, these might function as competing outcomes for slower or faster feed increases: intent to increase faster may result in more NEC, intent to increase slower may result in more LOS from longer indwelling catheter duration. The largest single trial to address this is the UK Speed of Increasing Feeds Trial (SIFT), recruiting 2,804 infants <32 weeks gestation or 1,500 g birth weight [18]. This RCT compared intention to feed at increases of 18 mL/kg/day with intention to feed at increases of 30 mL/kg/day. Importantly, infants were randomized once the clinician was comfortable increasing feeds and median age at increases commencing was 4 days (IQR 3–6). The primary outcome was survival without moderate or severe neurological impairment at 2 years of corrected gestational age, but predischarge morbidities including NEC and LOS were secondary outcomes, alongside a preplanned health economic evaluation. There were no statistically significant differences in predischarge morbidities or mortality. NEC occurred in 5% of the faster arm and 5.6% of the slower arm, culture positive LOS in 19.9% of the faster arm and 17.9% of the slower arm, and all LOS (including culture negative) in 30.1% of the faster arm and 27.5% of the slower arm. There was a difference of 2 days' duration of PN: median 7 days (IQR 7–10) for the faster arm, and 10 days (IQR 9–13) for the slower arm. This difference was statistically significant with an effect measure of 1.7 (95% CI 1.52–1.89) favoring faster feeds. At 2 years' correct-

ed gestational age, the primary was not statistically different: 65.5% (faster arm) and 68.1% (slower arm), effect measure 0.96 (95% CI 0.91–1.02). Subgroup analyses confirmed no impact of gestation on these findings, but motor impairment alone was different across the two arms, with more affected infants in the faster arm (7.5 vs. 5%), statistically significant at the 99% confidence level with a risk ratio of 1.48 (99% CI 1.02–2.14). There was no impact on the diagnosis of cerebral palsy, cognitive impairment, visual impairment, or hearing impairment. The possible mechanism behind motor impairment differences is unclear, and this effect may still be by chance. Overall, this very large study suggests that pragmatically approaching intent to increase "slower" or "faster," within the range 18–30 mL/kg/day does not impact on clinical outcome measures for most infants, but faster intent may shorten duration of PN. The accompanying health economic analysis suggested that faster feeding was more expensive by an average of GBP 267 per baby [19], resulting from the higher rates of adverse outcome even in the absence of statistical significance, arising from the stochastic approach to economic analysis as used by health decision maker groups such as the National Institute for Health and Clinical Excellence [20].

The 2017 Cochrane meta-analysis of slow versus fast feed increments [21] identified 9 studies of 3,576 infants (2,804 from SIFT). No difference was seen in mortality (OR 1.15 [95% CI 0.93–1.42]), NEC (OR 1.07 [95% CI 0.83–1.39]), or LOS (OR 1.15 [95% CI 1.0–1.32]). Clinical decision makers may feel reassured to feed at increments of 30 mL/kg/day in a baby tolerating this well, but also assured that for a less tolerant baby advancing more slowly does not cause obvious harm.

Route of Gastric Tube Placement
Feeding tubes may be placed into the stomach (gastric G) or positioned across the pylorus (jejunal J) and sited nasally (N) or orally (O), meaning there are at least four possible placements of feeding tubes in preterm infants. Data are limited on route of placement (<200 infants studied) but suggest no clear differences in growth or adverse events for NG or OG placement and that gastric feeding is preferable [22], and more physiological in terms of GI tract hormone promotion, gastric emptying, and achieving normal GI motility [23].

Intermittent or Continuous Feeding Strategies
Feed can be delivered by small boluses to mimic normal feeding patterns, or continuously. Studies show no differences in time to achieve full feeds, growth, or NEC rates [24], but only included small numbers of infants weighing <1,000 g. Studies undertaken in the subsequent 10 years have not changed current understanding of risks and benefits of intermittent or continuous strategies.

Milk Tolerance

When to Slow Down, Pause or Stop Enteral Feeds

Individual infants may have specific clinical factors that clinicians feel add uncertainty about whether to attempt to increase feed as for infants without such factors, or whether there should be deliberate intent to advance more slowly. These include a significant patent ductus arteriosus (PDA), inotrope receipt, blood transfusion, being small for gestational age (SGA), or the presence of abnormal dopplers (AREDF) antenatally.

Infant Factors

The ADEPT trial addressed AREDF and SGA from a "when to start" perspective, reassuring clinicians that delaying feeding was not necessary [14]. SIFT, comparing rates of increasing, recruited all infants regardless of growth restriction (18% of recruits <19th centile) or AREDF (15% recruits) [18]. Primary outcome subgroup analysis of the growth-restricted infants still showed no impact of speed of increment (OR 1.04 [95% CI 0.92–1.17]), suggesting that a similar approach in these infants as for other infants is sensible, although subgroup analyses lack power compared to whole study analysis. Meta-analysis of this subgroup of infants with either growth restriction, AREDF, or both was also undertaken [15] confirming no change in NEC risks with early or late introduction of feeds (OR for NEC 0.87 [95% CI 0.54–1.41]). There are less clear data for other infant factors: the number of infants needed for clinical end points (NEC or LOS) is often prohibitively large when subgroups of infants are considered. Some specific issues are considered below.

Blood Transfusion

Pausing feeding during packed red cell transfusion is advocated by some, given the reported association between transfusion and NEC and the observations of altered mesenteric flow during transfusion [25]. A pilot trial demonstrated feasibility of recruitment of infants to an electronic care record-based trial [26] and further data are awaited from ongoing trials.

Patent Ductus Arteriosus

Like PDA management itself, optimal feeding strategies for infants with a hemodynamically significant PDA are controversial, and opinions vary. Data on which to base decisions are limited: definitions of "significant" PDA are variable, as are definitions of feed tolerance, and full feeds. Current literature is reviewed in Martini et al. [27] but concludes with a caution around interpreting the current evidence as endorsing any one approach over another, rather encouraging an individualized hemodynamic based approach and calling for higher quality larger RCTs.

Feed Intolerance
Clinical thresholds for labelling an infant "'feed intolerant" are highly variable, often unit specific, and embedded in cultural practices, as evidenced by the large variation in TTF across the world [5]. Units may use a combination of stooling patterns, abdominal examination, abdominal girth, and gastric aspirates/residuals to label an infant "feed intolerant." Definitions of these issues are variable and non-standardized, making conclusions very difficult to draw.

Gastric Aspirate/Residuals

Gastric contents consist of milk (partially digested or undigested) and gastric secretions consisting of hormones, acid, and enzymes which aid digestion, promote GI motility, and intestinal maturation. Whilst discarding residual milk may not be harmful as long as volumes are replaced, discarding the associated components may be physiologically harmful [23], delay achievement of full enteral feeds, and reduce growth. Nonetheless, it is often practiced routinely in NICUs and difficult to stop. Studies assessing the impact of routine gastric aspiration found no differences in rates of NEC, but delayed time to regain birth weight was seen in one study of 80 infants with gastric aspiration in comparison to abdominal circumference measurement [28]. Larger studies are needed to definitively address this, with clinically relevant end points important to parents and infants.

Where gastric aspiration is undertaken, a further question is raised – what to do with the residual. A single trial has compared refeeding the residual to discarding and refeeding with fresh milk in infants between 23 and 28 weeks' gestation being fed by bolus feeds every 3 h [29], suggesting this appeared safe, but only 72 infants participated.

Monitoring

Unit Practices
Given the importance of the approach to early initiation and establishment of full enteral feeds, individual units are likely to benefit from agreed guidance to help staff share a similar approach. In addition, standardized feeding guidance has been shown to reduce the rates of NEC. As such, units would benefit from

monitoring through audit their own adherence to their feeding guidance, their actual TTF, and their use of PN.

Clinical Outcomes

Feed-associated outcomes are also important for individual units to understand their own data for, including rates of NEC, LOS, mortality, and 2 years' neurodevelopmental outcomes. These offer an ability to monitor outcomes over time and compare outcomes to similar units through systems like the Vermont Oxford Network (VON) or the UK National Neonatal Audit Programme (NNAP).

Individual Infant Monitoring

For individual infants, monitoring of the current feeding strategy is undertaken by a combination of biochemical and anthropometric measures. The importance of calcium and phosphorous in early feeding, the requirement for most preterm infants to be supplemented with sodium, vitamins, and minerals to adequately accrete tissue, and the immaturity of the preterm kidney makes regular biochemical monitoring essential. This should be supplemented with anthropometric monitoring to give a picture of body growth that is being achieved, although standards for this are subject to much discussion.

Mechanistic Monitoring

Given that the mechanisms linking feed approaches to outcomes such as NEC, LOS, and neurodevelopmental delay are incompletely understood, it is difficult to identify the best monitoring strategies for these elements. However, in the future it is possible that bedside microbial, metabolic, or inflammatory measures may be both much more routinely available, and more clearly mechanistically linked to outcomes, such that real time adjustments could be made. This may also apply to measures around breast milk content, such as routine monitoring of human milk oligosaccharide (HMO) content, IgA content, and potential modification of these elements, mechanistically linked to NEC [30]. Table 2 summarizes suggested monitoring strategies.

Summary and Suggestions for Future Research

This article summarizes the key practical steps in starting and increasing milk feeds, and a suggested approach to monitoring. As can be seen for some decisions, there are data on large numbers of infants supporting practice, but for others data are lacking or from small numbers of infants only. Moderate certainty exists around when to start, and a safe range in which to aim to progress

Table 2. Suggested monitoring strategies for early feed practices

Measure	Specifics	Relevance	Suggested comparator(s)
Clinical outcomes	NEC rates LOS rates 2-year neurodevelopmental outcomes Growth (change in z-scores)	Reflections of "success" of enteral feeding strategies	Year on year NNAP VON Other network
Unit practice (audits)	Time to full feeds Duration of PN % MOM first feed % MOM full feed % MOM at discharge	Measures of adherence to intent Ability to support MOM throughout feeding	Year on year NNAP VON Other network
Mechanisms of gut health	Stool microbiome Stool calprotectin MOM HMO profiles MOM sIgA	Potentially amenable to change through probiotic use, supplementation etc.	Literature-based profiles associated with "healthy" infants
Biochemistry	Serum electrolyte, bone profiles, vitamin and mineral levels	Amenable to supplementation	Reference ranges

milk feeds. Outcome measures in these studies are however usually very short term, and the emphasis is on rates of LOS and NEC, with the exception of SIFT, where 2-year outcome was the primary end point. Few studies focus on increasing receipt of maternal milk despite the clear benefits of this, and future studies should place more emphasis on the importance of receipt of maximal amounts of maternal milk. Mechanistic data obtained during feeding studies is also limited and may inform future study design and clinical practice.

Conflict of Interest Statement

J.E. Berrington declares research funding to her institution from Prolacta Biosciences and Danone Early Life Nutrition.

References

1 Granger CL, Embleton ND, Palmer JM, et al: Maternal breast milk, infant gut microbiome, and the impact on preterm infant health. Acta Paediatr. 2021;110:450–57.

2 Sherman MP, Zaghouani H and Niklas V: Gut microbiota, the immune system, and diet influence the neonatal gut-brain axis. Pediatr Res. 2015;77:127–35.

3 Bardanzellu F, Fanos V: How could metabolomics change pediatric health? Ital J Pediatr. 2020;46:37.

4 Wang M, Ivanov I, Davidson LA, et al: Infant nutrition and the microbiome: a systems biology approach to uncovering host-microbe interactions. In: Kussmann M, Stover P, editors. Nutrigenomics and Proteomics in Health and Disease: Towards a Systems Level Understanding of Gene Diet Interactions. London: Wylie and Sons; 2017.

5 de Waard M, Li Y, Zhu Y, et al: Time to full enteral feeding for very low-birth-weight infants varies markedly among hospitals worldwide but may not be associated with incidence of necrotizing enterocolitis: The NEOMUNE-NeoNutriNet Cohort Study. J Parenter Enter Nutr. 2019;43:658–67.

6 Webbe J, Brunton G, Ali S, et al: Parent, patient and clinician perceptions of outcomes during and following neonatal care: a systematic review of qualitative research. BMJ Paediatr Open. 2018;2:e000343.

7 Tao J, Mao J, Yang J, et al: Effects of oropharyngeal administration of colostrum on the incidence of necrotizing enterocolitis, late-onset sepsis, and death in preterm infants: a meta-analysis of RCTs. Eur J Clin Nutr. 2020;74:1122–131.

8 Sohn K, Kalanetra KM, Mills DA, et al: Buccal administration of human colostrum: impact on the oral microbiota of premature infants. J Perinatol. 2016;36:106–11.

9 Maffei D, Brewer M, Codipilly C, et al: Early oral colostrum administration in preterm infants. J Perinatol. 2020 Feb;40(2):284–87.

10 Lee J, Kim H-S, Jung YH, et al: Oropharyngeal colostrum administration in extremely premature infants: an RCT. Pediatrics. 2015;135:e357–66.

11 Snyder R, Herdt A, Mejias-Cepeda N, et al: Early provision of oropharyngeal colostrum leads to sustained breast milk feedings in preterm infants. Pediatr Neonatol. 2017;58:534–40.

12 Morgan J, Bombell S, Mcguire W: Early trophic feeding versus enteral fasting for very preterm or very low birth weight infants. Cochrane Database Syst Rev. 2013 Mar 28;(3):CD000504.

13 Mosqueda E, Sapiegiene L, Glynn L, et al: The early use of minimal enteral nutrition in extremely low birth weight newborns. J Perinatol. 2008;28:264–69.

14 Leaf A, Dorling J, Kempley S, et al: Early or delayed enteral feeding for preterm growth-restricted infants: a randomized trial. Pediatrics. 2012;129:e1260–e1268.

15 Morgan J, Young L, Mcguire W: Delayed introduction of progressive enteral feeds to prevent necrotising enterocolitis in very low birth weight infants. Cochrane Database Syst Rev. 2014;2014(12):CD001970.

16 Corpeleijn WE, Kouwenhoven SMP, Paap MC, et al: Intake of own mother's milk during the first days of life is associated with decreased morbidity and mortality in very low birth weight infants during the first 60 days of life. Neonatology. 2012;102:276–281.

17 Belfort MB, Anderson PJ, Nowak VA, et al: Breast milk feeding, brain development, and neurocognitive outcomes: a 7-year longitudinal study in infants born at less than 30 weeks' gestation. J Pediatr. 2016;177:133–139.e1.

18 Dorling J, Abbott J, Berrington J, et al: Controlled trial of two incremental milk-feeding rates in preterm infants. NEJM. 2019;381:1434–43.

19 Tahir W, Monahan M, Dorling J, et al: Economic evaluation alongside the Speed of Increasing milk Feeds Trial (SIFT). Arch Dis Child Fetal Neonatal Ed. 2020 Nov;105(6):587–92.

20 The National Institute for Health and Care: Guide to the Methods of Technology Appraisal. London: NICE; 2018. pp 1–93.

21 Oddie SJ, Young L, Mcguire W: Slow advancement of enteral feed volumes to prevent necrotising enterocolitis in very low birth weight infants. Cochrane Database Syst Rev. 2021 Aug;8(8):CD001241.

22 Watson J, Mcguire W: Transpyloric versus gastric tube feeding for preterm infants. Cochrane Database Syst Rev. 2013 Feb 28;2013(2):CD003487.

23 Parker L, Torrazza R, Li, Y, et al: Aspiration and evaluation of gastric residuals in the NICU: state of the science. J Perinat Neonatal Nurs. 2015;29:51–9.

24 Premji SS, Chessell L: Continuous nasogastric milk feeding versus intermittent bolus milk feeding for premature infants less than 1,500 g. Cochrane Database Syst Rev. 2011;11:CD001819.

25 Krimmel GA, Baker R, Yanowitz TD: Blood transfusion alters the superior mesenteric artery blood flow velocity response to feeding in premature infants. Am J Perinatol. 2009;26:99–106.

26 Gale C, Modi N, Jawad S, et al: The WHEAT pilot trial – With Holding Enteral feeds around packed red cell Transfusion to prevent necrotising enterocolitis in preterm neonates: a multicentre, electronic patient record (EPR), randomised controlled point-of-care pilot trial. BMJ Open. 2019;9:1–7.

27 Martini S, Aceti A, Galletti S, et al: To feed or not to feed: a critical overview of enteral feeding management and gastrointestinal complications in preterm neonates with a patent ductus arteriosus. Nutrients. 2020;12:83.

28 Kaur A, Kler N, Saluja S, et al: Abdominal circumference or gastric residual volume as measure of feed intolerance in VLBW infants. J Pediatr Gastroenterol Nutr. 2015;60:259–63.

29 Salas AA, Cuna A, Bhat R, et al: A randomised trial of re-feeding gastric residuals in preterm infants. Arch Dis Child Fetal Neonat Ed. 2015;100:F224–28.

30 Masi AC, Embleton ND, Lamb CA, et al: Human milk oligosaccharide DSLNT and gut microbiome in preterm infants predicts necrotising enterocolitis. Gut. 2020 Dec 16;gutjnl-2020-322771. doi: 10.1136/gutjnl-2020-322771.

Janet E. Berrington
Clinical and Translational Research Institute
Newcastle University
Newcastle upon Tyne NE2 4HH
UK
j.e.berrington@newcastle.ac.uk

Published online: May 10, 2022

Embleton ND, Haschke F, Bode L (eds): Strategies in Neonatal Care to Promote Optimized Growth and Development: Focus on Low Birth Weight Infants. 96th Nestlé Nutrition Institute Workshop, May 2021. Nestlé Nutr Inst Workshop Ser. Basel, Karger, 2022, vol 96, pp 13–22 (DOI: 10.1159/000519391)

Strategies in Neonatal Care to Promote Growth and Neurodevelopment of the Preterm Infant

Frank H. Bloomfield[a]   Barbara E. Cormack[a, b]

[a]Liggins Institute, University of Auckland, Auckland, New Zealand; [b]Starship Child Health, Auckland City Hospital, Auckland, New Zealand

Abstract

Recommendations for nutrition of very preterm and very low birth weight infants have developed over time with our understanding of the requirements of preterm babies and the awareness of widespread poor postnatal growth. In general, the trend has been towards enhancing nutrition, but more recent recommendations have begun to raise questions with respect to the potential for high and early nutritional intakes, particularly of protein, to carry risks such as refeeding syndrome. However, large gaps in our knowledge remain for both macro- and micronutrient requirements to support optimal growth and how nutrition and growth relate to important long-term outcomes. Closing these knowledge gaps has been hampered by inconsistent reporting of nutrition intakes and growth parameters, small trials with short-term outcomes and the use of a variety of different methods of monitoring growth. The challenge now is for future research to address these issues through consensus building around the important questions that need to be answered, how to report data from neonatal nutritional trials and whether large trials answering important questions can take place through development of consortia that undertake similar trials in multiple jurisdictions with agreements to share data.   © 2022 S. Karger AG, Basel

Supporting growth of preterm newborns, particularly those born very or extremely preterm, through regular monitoring on growth charts and careful attention to their nutrition is consistent with all pediatric practice, measuring growth of all children as surveillance for failure to thrive, malnutrition, or stunting. Why then, do we still not understand what the optimal growth trajectory is for these vulnerable babies nor have consensus on how we should measure them? Until recently, the generally accepted recommendation was that preterm babies should grow along a trajectory similar to that of the fetus. Yet we know that preterm babies, as a population, are born growth-restricted compared with their gestational-age-matched intrauterine peers who go on to be born at term. We use weight as a proxy for growth and we plot growth on cross-sectional charts of birth weight. The driver for promoting growth is that better in-hospital growth is associated with better neurodevelopmental outcome. The assumption follows that better nutrition will lead to better growth and, therefore, better neurodevelopmental outcomes, but high-quality evidence to support this assumption is lacking.

Measuring Growth

Weight is a measure of mass, not of growth. Increases in mass can be due to true growth of lean mass or accumulation of fluid or other tissue, such as fat or pathological tissue. To assess growth requires measurement of length (in babies, rather than height). In babies, head circumference correlates well with brain growth, so measurement of head circumference also is a useful measure, although the potential impact of short-term changes due to molding of head shape from lying position or from equipment used to secure continuous positive airway pressure systems needs to be borne in mind. There are numerous length boards and neonatometers now available that fit easily into incubators and non-stretch head circumference tapes that make measurement of length and head circumference on a regular basis (e.g., weekly) relatively straightforward. Regular measurement of all three parameters should be routine practice in neonatal intensive care and smooths out the inevitable inaccuracies due to the challenges that exist in measuring sick preterm infants reliably and consistently. More precise measurement of linear growth, accurate to a magnitude of change similar to 1–2 days' linear growth, can be obtained for research purposes using a knemometer [1].

Bloomfield/Cormack

Monitoring Growth

When plotting preterm babies' size at birth on cross-sectional growth charts, the distribution approximates a Gaussian distribution, but when plotted on fetal growth charts the distribution is skewed to the left, demonstrating that, as a population, preterm babies are growth restricted [2]. Fetal growth trajectory is associated with gestation length [3]. However, fetal ultrasound charts do not include length or head circumference, meaning they are not useful for the postnatal monitoring of growth.

Thus, postnatal growth needs to be measured on postnatal growth charts. Most of these are cross-sectional charts based on the birth weight of babies across the gestational age spectrum. The INTERGROWTH-21st consortium has published postnatal longitudinal growth charts for "healthy" preterm babies, but includes only 201 babies, 12 of whom were born very preterm (27–32 weeks' gestation, with none below 27 weeks) [4]. Large numbers of different birth weight centile charts for preterm babies are available and are used in reporting growth outcomes [5]. This makes comparing growth across studies very challenging, as the same baby plotted on different charts could be interpreted as having very different outcomes. For example, a baby born at 27 weeks with a birth weight that sits on the 10th percentile on the UK-WHO growth charts and who then grows along the 10th percentile on the UK-WHO growth charts (with a z-score change of zero from birth to term-corrected age) will demonstrate a decrease of approximately one z-score when plotted on the Fenton growth charts and a drop of 1.2 standard deviations on the INTERGROWTH-21st postnatal growth charts (Fig. 1). An alternative to describing postnatal growth according to z-score change, at least until there is consensus on which chart should be used, is to describe the actual change in growth as an incremental change, for example grams per day or grams per kilogram per day. The latter is more robust, taking into account the size of the baby (similar incremental growth can be calculated for length and head circumference), but does not account for different growth velocities across the gestational age spectrum nor for sex. There remains debate about how best incremental change in growth should be calculated [5, 6]. Given the fact that all babies lose weight after birth (see below), should birth weight be used as a reference point, the minimum weight before weight-gain starts again or a fixed point in time when babies are expected to have stabilized their weight [7]? All of the above have been proposed, and there are reasonable arguments for each, but clearly the reference point taken will impact upon the assessment of subsequent growth trajectory and, therefore, potentially the identification of faltering postnatal growth. Once a reference has been determined, there also are differences in the method used to calculate growth velocity, the three most common being: net weight gain over time interval divided by the time interval

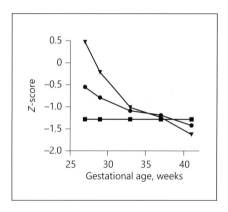

Fig. 1. Z-score change for length from birth to discharge differs according to growth chart used. Length of a boy born at 27 weeks' gestation is plotted on the UK-WHO (■), Fenton 2013 [29] (●), and INTERGROWTH-21st [4] (▼) growth charts. Linear growth would be considered appropriate according to the UK-WHO charts as there is no change in z-score but faltering according to the Fenton 2013 (a decrease of 0.9 z-score) and INTERGROWTH-21st (a decrease of 1.2 z-score) charts. Differences below 30 weeks' postmenstrual age are likely due to more recent data with better estimation of gestational age and a substantially larger sample size in the Fenton data (Fenton, $n = 12{,}000$ and UK-WHO, $n = 146$ less than 30 weeks' gestation; INTERGROWTH-21st, $n = 12$ born less than 32 weeks' gestation). Differences near term are likely to be due to the smoothing of the Fenton charts from prenatal growth to postnatal growth data, taking account of the slowing of intrauterine growth near term that one would not expect to see in preterm babies at the same corrected gestational age.

and starting weight; net weight gain over time interval divided by the time interval and the mean of starting weight and weight at the time of interest, and an exponential method. These different methods can result in substantial differences in estimated weight gain in $g \times kg^{-1} \times day^{-1}$ with potential impact on nutritional decisions [5, 6].

Compounding the interpretation of postnatal growth is the tendency to use the term "extrauterine growth failure" to mean a baby's position on a growth chart at a particular point in time, for example, a baby below the 10th percentile at 36 weeks' postmenstrual age or at term-corrected age [8]. This, clearly, is a nonsense as an individual's position on the chart will be determined in a large part by the starting position of that individual and growth faltering is predicated upon a change in velocity, not on a static point in time. A baby born at or below the 10th percentile and who is just below the 10th percentile at term-corrected age is likely to have had perfectly adequate growth.

Furthermore, all babies lose weight after birth due to loss of extracellular fluid, and Rochow et al. [9] have demonstrated that, when plotted on the Fenton growth charts, this loss appears to stabilize at approximately –0.8 standard deviation (z) scores regardless of gestation. However, of note is that for very preterm babies, one standard deviation around the mean extends from a weight loss of approximately –0.4 to –1.2 z-scores, indicating that 17% of very preterm babies have a decrease in z-score for weight of greater than –1.2. Shifts in fluid and the effects of molding may also affect head circumference measurements after birth, and there is some evidence to indicate that linear growth also slows around birth, at least following vaginal birth, but these changes have not been quantified reliably for preterm babies and may be relatively greater than for term birth due to the stress associated with preterm birth [10].

To advance our ability to interpret growth of preterm babies and the impact of different growth trajectories on important outcomes, it is essential to be able to compare results of different research. To be able to do so, we need consensus on, at a minimum, the following: growth charts to be used for plotting growth; method of calculating postnatal growth velocity; the definition of postnatal faltering growth, and the growth variables to be reported.

Growth and Long-Term Outcome

The underlying reason for monitoring postnatal growth is to ensure that growth is adequate to support optimal neurodevelopment without adverse effects, such as excess accumulation of fat or later increased risk of adverse metabolic outcomes. For example, in preterm babies more rapid linear growth between term-corrected age and 4 months has been associated with decreased odds at age 8 years of an intelligence quotient more than one standard deviation below the mean (odds ratio [OR] and 95% confidence intervals [CI] 0.82 [0.70–0.96] per 1 z-score increase in linear growth), but increased odds of overweight or obesity (OR 1.27 [1.05–1.53]) [11].

Most studies report a positive association between in-hospital growth of extremely preterm babies and long-term neurodevelopmental outcome (for example, see [12]), but this does not imply causation. Preterm babies that have a straightforward course are likely to both grow better and to have better neurodevelopmental outcomes. As might be expected from the discussion above, the association between growth and outcome will depend upon the methods of determining growth and the definitions used to define adequate growth or growth faltering. Recent data from follow-up of a randomized controlled trial indicate that poor postnatal growth, defined as a decline in growth trajectory above a threshold, determined using fetal growth charts (that is, those using cross-sectional data from size at birth) may be a better predictor of poor neurodevelopmental outcomes than poor postnatal growth determined using the longitudinal INTERGROWTH charts [13], but more data are needed.

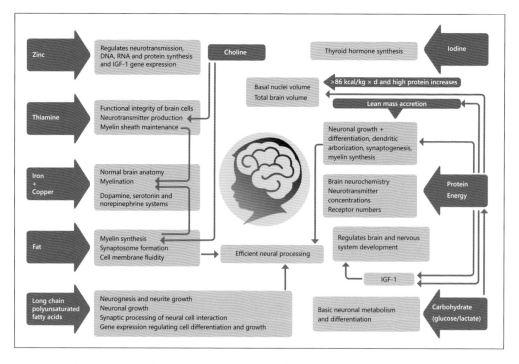

Fig. 2. Schematic of nutrients required for brain growth and development. Reproduced from Cormack et al. [30] (available at https://doi.org/10.3390/nu11092029) under the terms of the Creative Commons Attribution License (http://creativecommons.org/licenses/by/4.0/).

Nutrition, Growth and Long-Term Outcome

In fetal life, growth is determined by nutrition; after birth, growth is determined by genes providing nutrition is sufficient. Multiple components of nutrition are required to support brain growth and development (Fig. 2). Breast milk composition is highly variable, but when given at 150 mL × kg^{-1} × day^{-1}, a common upper limit for enteral feeds, the macronutrient content, particularly of protein, is unlikely to be sufficient to support adequate growth. Additional macronutrients are, therefore, often provided as supplements to breast milk, either as multicomponent fortifiers or as single macronutrient supplements. Cochrane meta-analyses suggest that these do result in increased in-hospital growth, including linear and head circumference growth, but the quality of evidence is low, and there are no data on long-term outcomes [14, 15]. Recent meta-analyses of trials that have provided nutritional supplementation (including enriched infant formula) to babies born preterm or small-for-gestational-age found that in toddlers

(<3 years of age; 29–31 trials, 2,797–2,924 toddlers) supplementation increased weight (mean difference [95% confidence intervals (CI)] 0.16 [0.01–0.30] kg), and length/height (mean difference 0.44 [0.10–0.77] cm), but not head circumference (mean difference 0.15 [–0.03 to 0.33] cm), with a subgroup analysis of 2 trials (173 boys, 159 girls) finding an effect in boys but not girls [16]. There were no consistent effects through later childhood, adolescence, or in adulthood. Similarly, there were no effects on cognitive scores or cognitive impairment (21 trials, 3,680 infants), although once again subgroup analyses suggested that toddler boys, but not girls, may have small benefits in cognitive scores [17]. There also were no effects on motor scores, although fewer supplemented children had motor impairment (relative risk [RR] 0.76 [0.62–0.94]) [17]. These possible effects on cognitive scores in boys and for motor impairment did not persist through to childhood, although the number of children included is much smaller. The meta-analysis concluded that overall quality of evidence is low to very low; an individual participant data meta-analysis is underway [18].

Similarly, a meta-analysis of trials investigating higher versus lower parenteral amino acid intakes in preterm babies found a reduction in postnatal growth failure (defined as weight <10th percentile at discharge, RR 0.74 [0.56–0.97]) but insufficient evidence to assess impact on long-term neurodevelopmental outcomes [19]. Quality of evidence was very low, and there are several more recent trials not included in this meta-analysis.

In summary, trials of enhanced nutrition, or of nutritional supplementation, in preterm and small-for-gestational-age babies have, in general, focused on short-term outcomes, are mostly of small size, and provide low-quality evidence, with very few trials addressing outcomes that are truly important, such as survival free from neurodisability or childhood metabolic/cardiovascular health as the primary outcome.

Concerns also have been raised that providing enhanced nutrition to sick, preterm babies may be harmful [20]. Although most studies have found a positive association between nutrition and growth, some have reported decreased measures of growth [21, 22]. A further potential concern of enhanced nutrition is the risk of refeeding syndrome, a biochemical disturbance characterized by hypophosphatemia, hypokalemia, and hypercalcemia, which may arise upon refeeding malnourished individuals [23, 24]. As discussed above, as a population preterm babies are growth restricted, and many may have been exposed to relative undernutrition due to placental dysfunction. Refeeding syndrome has been reported to occur in a significant proportion of extremely preterm babies, to be associated with nutritional intakes, and with clinical outcomes [24]. However, refeeding syndrome appears to be more complex than simply being related to higher protein and energy intakes as, in a large, multicenter, prospective cohort study, the incidence of refeeding syndrome varied widely amongst centers, and some centers with higher protein and energy intakes reported lower incidences of refeeding syndrome [24].

In general, the current approach is to provide nutrition, particularly enteral nutrition, early to extremely preterm infants because of their minimal stores, rapid growth phase and to avoid an accumulating nitrogen deficit. However, findings from the PEPaNIC randomized trial in pediatric intensive care units [25], which compared withholding parenteral nutrition (PN) for 1 week with early (before 24–48 h) initiation of PN, raised concerns about whether early provision of PN is appropriate in preterm babies. A preplanned secondary subgroup analysis of the PEPaNIC trial of critically ill term neonates ($n = 209$) in pediatric intensive care found that late initiation increased the likelihood of live discharge from pediatric intensive care (hazard ratio 1.61 [1.19–2.20]) [26]. In neonates aged up to 1 week ($n = 145$), the risk of infection was reduced with late initiation of PN (adjusted odds ratio 0.36 [0.15–0.83]) [26]. At 2-year follow-up of the whole PEPaNIC cohort (mean age at follow-up approximately 6 years), executive function as reported by the parent or caregiver was reported to be improved in children who had received late initiation of PN [27].

There has been extensive commentary on the PEPaNIC trial and its implications for preterm babies given that there were no preterm babies included in the trial. A key concern is the provision of energy intakes in excess of recommendations in the early group and substantially higher than in the late group. Overfeeding is potentially harmful, and there were no reports of biochemistry data, meaning it is not possible to determine whether refeeding syndrome in the early group was a significant factor. The PEPaNIC trial findings therefore need to inform future research in preterm infants, rather than influencing current practice. Results from the ProVIDe trial, a multicenter, triple-blind randomized controlled trial of an additional $1 \text{ g} \times \text{d}^{-1}$ of amino acids for the first 5 days after birth on survival free from neurodisability at 2 years of age [28] should provide valuable information on whether similar risks of enhanced early nutrition may apply to extremely preterm babies.

Conclusions

Nutrition for very preterm babies is a universal, relatively simple, and inexpensive part of their care, yet we still do not understand what a package of nutritional support that will provide optimal long-term outcomes looks like. Progress has been hampered by small trials, often with methodological weaknesses, with short-term outcomes and inconsistency of reporting of key outcomes of interest.

Future research should identify priorities for research that need to be developed through a robust prioritization framework including families, standardization of reporting through the development of Core Outcome and Minimal Reporting Sets for nutritional studies in preterm infants, and the development of international consortia to undertake trials that, when combined through meta-analysis and, ideally, individual participant data meta-analysis, are large enough to address important outcomes.

Conflict of Interest Statement

Professor Frank Bloomfield is Director of the Liggins Institute at the University of Auckland. Dr. Barbara Cormack is a Nestlé Nutrition Institute Oceania Paediatric Advisory Board Member.

References

1 Gibson AT, Pearse RG, Wales JK. Knemometry and the assessment of growth in premature babies. Arch Dis Child. 1993;69(5):498–504.

2 Cooke RW. Conventional birth weight standards obscure fetal growth restriction in preterm infants. Arch Dis Child Fetal Neonatal Ed. 2007;92(3):F189–92.

3 Lackman F, Capewell V, Richardson B, et al. The risks of spontaneous preterm delivery and perinatal mortality in relation to size at birth according to fetal versus neonatal growth standards. Am J Obstet Gynecol. 2001;184(5):946–53.

4 Villar J, Giuliani F, Bhutta ZA, et al. Postnatal growth standards for preterm infants: the Preterm Postnatal Follow-up Study of the INTER-GROWTH-21(st) Project. Lancet Glob Health. 2015 Nov;3(11):e681–91.

5 Cormack BE, Embleton ND, van Goudoever JB, et al. Comparing apples with apples: it is time for standardized reporting of neonatal nutrition and growth studies. Pediatr Res. 2016;79(6):810–20.

6 Fenton TR, Griffin IJ, Hoyos A, et al. Accuracy of preterm infant weight gain velocity calculations vary depending on method used and infant age at time of measurement. Pediatr Res. 2019;85(5):650–54.

7 Fenton TR, Chan HT, Madhu A, et al. Preterm infant growth velocity calculations: a systematic review. Pediatrics 2017;139(3):e20162045.

8 Fenton TR, Cormack B, Goldberg D, et al. "Extra-uterine growth restriction" and "postnatal growth failure" are misnomers for preterm infants. J Perinatol. 2020;40(5):704–14.

9 Rochow N, Raja P, Liu K, et al. Physiological adjustment to postnatal growth trajectories in healthy preterm infants. Pediatr Res. 2016;79(6):870–9.

10 Teele RL, Abbott GD, Mogridge N, Teele DW. Femoral growth lines: bony birthmarks in infants. Am J Roentgenol. 1999;173(3):719–22.

11 Belfort MB, Gillman MW, Buka SL, et al. Preterm infant linear growth and adiposity gain: trade-offs for later weight status and intelligence quotient. J Pediatr. 2013;163(6):1564–69 e2.

12 Hickey L, Burnett A, Spittle AJ, et al. Extreme prematurity, growth and neurodevelopment at 8 years: a cohort study. Arch Dis Child. 2021;106(2):160–66.

13 Cordova EG, Cherkerzian S, Bell K, et al. Association of poor postnatal growth with neurodevelopmental impairment in infancy and childhood: comparing the fetus and the healthy preterm infant references. J Pediatr. 2020;225:37–43 e5.

14 Brown JV, Embleton ND, Harding JE, McGuire W. Multi-nutrient fortification of human milk for preterm infants. Cochrane Database Syst Rev. 2016;8(5):CD000343.

15 Amissah EA, Brown J, Harding JE. Protein supplementation of human milk for promoting growth in preterm infants. Cochrane Database Syst Rev. 2020 Sep 23;9:CD000433.

16 Lin L, Amissah E, Gamble GD, et al. Impact of macronutrient supplements on later growth of children born preterm or small for gestational age: a systematic review and meta-analysis of randomised and quasirandomised controlled trials. PLoS Med. 2020;17(5):e1003122.

17 Lin L, Amissah E, Gamble GD, et al. Impact of macronutrient supplements for children born preterm or small for gestational age on developmental and metabolic outcomes: a systematic review and meta-analysis. PLoS Med. 2019;16(10):e1002952.

18 Lin L, Crowther C, Gamble G, et al. Sex-specific effects of nutritional supplements in infants born early or small: protocol for an individual participant data meta-analysis (ESSENCE IPD-MA). BMJ Open. 2020;8;10(1):e033438.

19 Osborn DA, Schindler T, Jones LJ, et al. Higher versus lower amino acid intake in parenteral nutrition for newborn infants. Cochrane Database Syst Rev. 2018;3(3):CD005949.

20 Modi N. The implications of routine milk fortification for the short and long-term health of preterm babies. Semin Fetal Neonatal Med. 2021 Jun;26(3):101216.

21 Blanco CL, Gong AK, Schoolfield J, et al. Impact of early and high amino acid supplementation on ELBW infants at 2 years. J Pediatr Gastroenterol Nutr. 2012;54(5):601–7.

22 Uthaya S, Liu X, Babalis D, et al. Nutritional Evaluation and Optimisation in Neonates: a randomized, double-blind controlled trial of amino acid regimen and intravenous lipid composition in preterm parenteral nutrition. Am J Clin Nutr. 2016;103(6):1443–52.

23 Moltu SJ, Strommen K, Blakstad EW, et al. Enhanced feeding in very-low-birth-weight infants may cause electrolyte disturbances and septicemia – a randomized, controlled trial. Clin Nutr. 2013;32(2):207–12.

24 Cormack BE, Jiang Y, Harding JE, et al. Neonatal refeeding syndrome and clinical outcome in extremely low-birth-weight babies: secondary cohort analysis from the ProVIDe trial. JPEN J Parenter Enteral Nutr. 2021;45(1):65–78.

25 Fivez T, Kerklaan D, Mesotten D, et al. Early versus late parenteral nutrition in critically ill children. N Engl J Med. 2016;374(12):1111–22.

26 van Puffelen E, Vanhorebeek I, Joosten KFM, et al. Early versus late parenteral nutrition in critically ill, term neonates: a preplanned secondary subgroup analysis of the PEPaNIC multicentre, randomised controlled trial. Lancet Child Adolesc Health. 2018;2(7):505–15.

27 Verstraete S, Verbruggen SC, Hordijk JA, et al. Long-term developmental effects of withholding parenteral nutrition for 1 week in the paediatric intensive care unit: a 2-year follow-up of the PEPaNIC international, randomised, controlled trial. Lancet Respir Med. 2019;7(2):141–53.

28 Bloomfield FH, Crowther CA, Harding JE, et al. The ProVIDe study: the impact of protein intravenous nutrition on development in extremely low birthweight babies. BMC Pediatr. 2015;15:100.

29 Fenton TR, Kim JH. A systematic review and meta-analysis to revise the Fenton growth chart for preterm infants. BMC Pediatr. 2013;13:59.

30 Cormack BE, Harding JE, Miller SP, Bloomfield FH. The influence of early nutrition on brain growth and neurodevelopment in extremely preterm babies: a narrative review. Nutrients. 2019 Aug;11(9):2029.

Frank H. Bloomfield
Liggins Institute
University of Auckland
Auckland 1142
New Zealand
f.bloomfield@auckland.ac.nz

Published online: May 10, 2022

Embleton ND, Haschke F, Bode L (eds): Strategies in Neonatal Care to Promote Optimized Growth and Development: Focus on Low Birth Weight Infants. 96th Nestlé Nutrition Institute Workshop, May 2021. Nestlé Nutr Inst Workshop Ser. Basel, Karger, 2022, vol 96, pp 23–33 (DOI: 10.1159/000519389)

Nutritional Interventions to Improve Brain Outcomes in Preterm Infants

Nicholas D. Embleton[a, b]   Claire Granger[a, c]
Kristina Chmelova[a, b]

[a]Newcastle Hospitals NHS Foundation Trust, Newcastle upon Tyne, UK; [b]Population Health Sciences Institute, Newcastle University, Newcastle upon Tyne, UK; [c]Translational and Clinical Research Institute, Newcastle University, Newcastle upon Tyne, UK

Abstract

The last 20 years have seen dramatic improvements in survival for preterm infants in both high- and low-income settings. Survival rates of over 50% in infants born 16 weeks early (24 weeks' gestation) are now commonplace in well-resourced neonatal intensive care units. However, ensuring adequate nutrient intakes especially in the first few days and weeks is challenging, and many infants show poor growth and nutritional status. Good nutritional management should be seen as the cornerstone of good neonatal care and is key to improving a range of important outcomes including reduced rates of retinopathy of prematurity, chronic lung disease, necrotizing enterocolitis (NEC), and sepsis. Equally importantly, is that good nutritional status is essential to optimize brain growth and differentiation. There are multiple potential mechanisms that link nutrition to brain outcomes in preterm infants including needs for tissue accretion, energy supply, signaling roles, functional components in human milk, epigenetic regulation, prevention of NEC and disease, and impacts on the gut brain axes. This article will review data in support of different mechanistic links for the impact of nutrition on brain outcomes in preterm infants.   © 2022 S. Karger AG, Basel

Introduction

Neonatal care has progressed rapidly in the last 20–30 years, and survival at 24 weeks gestation is now common in well-resourced settings. Neonatal care expanded rapidly in the 1960s and 1970s, yet in the early days practice on neonatal intensive care units (NICUs) was focused on cardiorespiratory care. The next few decades showed dramatic decreases in death from respiratory distress syndrome and other complications; however, there was a general lack of focus on nutrition. Whilst parenteral nutrition (PN) has been available for neonates since the last 1960s, it was rarely used routinely for preterm infants until the 1990s. Similarly, whilst the importance of human milk (HM) for promoting lifelong health has always been recognized [1], many NICUs start enteral feeds quite slowly meaning exposure to the benefits of HM are limited in the first few days. Preterm infants present many challenges to achieving adequate nutrition. This includes metabolic intolerance, for example hyperglycemia, hypophosphatemia, etc. during PN, and enteral tolerance, which results in many preterm infants not achieving full enteral milk volumes until around day 10–14. Even at this stage, where "full" milk feed volumes of around 150–180 mL/kg/day are achieved, the relatively low macronutrient density of HM means full milk feeds do not equate to achieving adequate macronutrient intakes [2]. A lack of focus on nutritional management in the first few days and weeks, combined with challenges in providing both PN and enteral nutrition mean that postnatal malnutrition remains universal in many NICUs [3]. Unfortunately, signs of malnutrition are not easy to see in the first few days. Thereafter, growth (most often assessed simply by weight gain) is often slower than fetal references. Whilst there is a robust and appropriate debate about optimal weight gain in preterm infants, it is clear to most healthcare practitioners (HCPs) that suboptimal nutritional management is common. Nutrient intakes rarely meet needs in the first few days and weeks resulting in poor growth that is associated with worse longer-term outcomes, especially suboptimal neuro-cognitive function.

Optimizing Nutritional Status

Whilst all HCPs recognize the importance of good nutrition, detailed knowledge of mechanisms and requirements tends to be restricted to those with specialized knowledge, and many clinicians lack a conceptual framework for assessing nutrition. Indeed, many HCPs tend to focus primarily on nutrient intakes without always appreciating the wider aspects that are needed to form a holistic assessment of nutrition for that infant. Nutritional practice includes the following areas:

1. *Macronutrient and micronutrient intakes*: whilst there is a lack of randomized controlled trials (RCTs) to determine optimal intakes for most nutrients, expert consensus guidelines provide details of recommended intakes that are widely accepted [4].

2. *Functional components*: most nutrients provided in PN and formula milk simply provide nutrients for tissue accretion or act as an energy source although even in these relatively "simple" fluids there are components that have wider functional activities such as prebiotics and certain amino acids (e.g., taurine and glutamine). However, these are dwarfed by the huge multitude of functional components provided in HM such as HM oligosaccharides (HMOs), growth factors such as IGF-1, and hormones such as insulin, none of which are in formula milk [5].

3. *Microbiomic aspects*: the last 10 years have seen a huge increase in research on gut microbiota that demonstrate the dramatic impact gut microbes have on mortality and morbidity (such as necrotizing enterocolitis, NEC) in preterm infants. Newborn infants are born relatively free of microbes but must rapidly develop immune tolerance against hundreds of microbial species. Gut microbial community composition is affected by the quantity and quality of enteral intakes, i.e. human versus cow milk, as well as the specific composition of HM [6], and supplements such as breast milk fortifiers and iron. In turn, gut microbes produce compounds essential for health such as vitamins, short-chain fatty acids and amino acids, as well as being involved in bile acid metabolism. Gut microbial composition is therefore integral to nutritional health.

4. *Socio-behavioral and technical aspects*: attitudes and behaviors of HCPs and use of donor HM (DHM) affect whether mothers continue to produce mother's own milk (MOM) [7], use of nasogastric tubes impacts on upper gastrointestinal microbial colonization, and delivery of milk using continuous, or bolus feeds impacts on gastric emptying, gall bladder emptying, and nutrient absorption.

Considering these different elements, the goal of nutritional management in preterm infants is to optimize nutritional status rather than simply maximize weight gain. Nutritional status in turn, is determined by:

1. What happened in the past, i.e. fetal growth restriction, maternal nutritional status such as vitamin D concentration, or previous disease, for example NEC.

2. Present body composition and metabolic tolerance, i.e. an infant's ability to tolerate a carbohydrate load, or dispose of excess amino acids (autophagy), as well as enteral/gastrointestinal tolerance, e.g. gastric emptying, intestinal motility, etc.

3. Desired future outcomes: whilst growth on the NICU is the most tangible evidence of nutritional intakes, later life outcomes such as metabolic disease and neurocognitive outcome are far more important and relevant to life-long health.

These three components combine to affect the ideal nutritional management for an individual baby that will optimize overall nutritional status. An infant with good nutritional status will demonstrate appropriate weight gain, with acceptable body composition, be able to tolerate nutrient intakes to meet needs and have high intakes of functional components from HM that enable the infant to optimize long-term brain outcomes.

Brain Growth and Nutrition in Early Life

Humans differ from other mammals by having a very large brain which is responsible for around 60–70% of all energy expenditure in early infant life. Between 24 weeks gestation and 2 years of age, humans acquire about 85–90% of the final adult volume. More importantly however, there are multiple overlapping neurological processes that take place in a time-coordinated fashion in early life (Fig. 1) [8, 9]. Throughout all three trimesters of pregnancy, neuronal migration is critical for development of all brain regions. During the 2nd and 3rd trimesters, apoptosis (programmed cell death) is particularly active but continues post-term into early infancy. Synaptogenesis is especially active during the 3rd trimester, throughout infancy, and into early childhood, and myelination that starts in the 3rd trimester does not complete until the 2nd decade of life. The impact of nutrient deficiency depends on which nutrient is involved (depicted in Figure 1 by theoretical nutrients A, B, C), the amount of the deficit (represented by the height of the box in Figure 1), and the timing and duration. A large but short-lived deficit of nutrient A (for example protein in first few days) will result in a different long-term neurocognitive phenotype to nutrient C where the deficit occurs later, is less severe, but lasts longer (for example choline). There are strong data to show that IGF-1 and other growth factors are responsible for brain growth and differentiation in early life. Recent data also show that IGF-1 concentrations are linked to brain growth in preterm infants [10]. Of major concern is that IGF-1 concentrations are frequently lower in preterm infants than those observed in utero or in newborn infants born full term. Further studies are needed, but there are some data to show that IGF-1 concentrations may be related to macronutrient intakes, emphasizing the importance of meeting nutrient needs in the NICU.

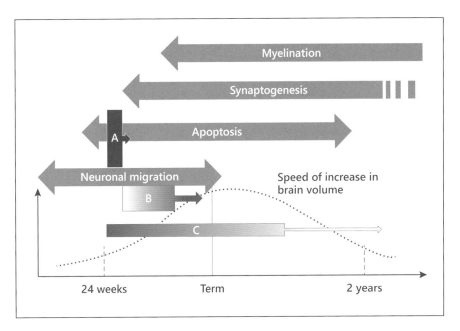

Fig. 1. Brain growth and nutrient deficits in preterm infants. Speed of increase in brain volume on *y* axis, depicted by blue dotted line and four developmental processes shown by grey arrow bars. A, B and C represent three theoretical nutrients that impact on brain growth and development. The longer-term neurocognitive phenotype will differ depending on the amount (height of box), type, timing, and duration (box and arrow) of any deficit in nutrient supply.

Placental nutrient transfer, fetal growth, duration of pregnancy, and composition of breastmilk evolved over millennia to optimize brain growth at different stages in the first 1,000 days of life. Human physiology aims to maximize survival with good brain outcomes, even if this is at the expense of later metabolic risk. In full-term infants, there is strong evidence of a dose-response effect of HM intakes on longer-term brain outcomes. Except at the extremes, however, there is relatively little evidence that growth or weight gain per se in healthy infants impacts on brain outcomes, unless slow growth is accompanied by specific nutrient deficiencies such as iron or iodine. Healthy full-term babies optimize long-term neurocognitive outcomes by receiving HM for as long as possible, largely independent of how quickly they gain weight. In contrast, there are good observational data linking growth to later brain outcomes, that are supported by a small number of RCTs in preterm infants. However, it is critical to appreciate that "faster" growth itself does not cause better brain outcomes. In fact, growth is simply a marker of good nutritional status rather than weight gain being on the causative pathway to brain growth. Weight gain is a reliable indicator of nutrient intakes in preterm infants, but there will always be individual variation, and it is impossible to know the optimal rate of weight gain for an individual. HM-fed infants on the NICU tend to gain weight more slowly than those receiving artificial formula; however, HM-fed infants will have better brain and metabolic outcomes. This has been termed the so-called "breastfeeding paradox," although many would consider there is nothing very paradoxical about nutrients of higher quality resulting in better outcomes [11].

One Brain for Life

Preterm infants have "one brain for life," and every aspect of clinical practice on the NICU should aim to protect and promote brain development. Preterm infants have very high nutrient requirements per kg bodyweight and are prone to macro- and micronutrient deficiencies due to low stores. Furthermore, they frequently lack the metabolic capacity to convert essential nutrients into functional components, meaning some nutrients that are not typically considered to be essential, become essential or conditionally essential such as certain fatty and amino acids. Aside from "nutritional" aspects of brain vulnerability, direct damage to the brain as evidenced by intraventricular hemorrhage or cystic periventricular leukomalacia is common in preterm infants. Whilst there are no data to suggest that typical nutritional management can directly prevent these complications, there are good reasons to think that nutritional management can impact on long-term outcome if these conditions have occurred. Very few RCTs have explored the impact of nutritional interventions specifically in high-risk infants with evidence of "brain damage," but there are some data to show that higher intakes of macronutrients post-discharge may improve outcome [12]. There are also limited data to suggest that supplementation with docosahexaenoic acid (DHA) and choline may improve neurocognitive outcomes, but large confirmatory trials are needed [13].

The poor neurocognitive outcome of babies who develop NEC has been well documented, but the precise mechanisms are likely to be multifactorial [14]. Most importantly, the associated "cytokine storm" activates cell surface receptors in the brain, especially Toll-like receptors on the surface of microglial cells, that trigger downstream release of inflammatory and pro-oxidant compounds that damage the cell [15]. Whilst there is no data to suggest that specific nutrients could prevent or modulate this process per se, there is (1) strong evidence that NEC is related to gut microbial patterns which are themselves modulated by dietary exposures [6] and (2) strong evidence that NEC is less common in infants receiving MOM. Therefore, there are mechanisms that link nutrition to disease prevention and thereby better brain outcomes. Providing HM nutrition therefore improves brain outcomes by preventing disease.

Macronutrient and Human Milk Intakes and Later Brain Outcome

Whilst there are few RCTs specifically focused on infants with radiological evidence of brain damage, there are several RCTs of "enhanced" nutrition in more typical populations of preterm infants that show better short- and longer-term brain outcomes. Studies show that greater macronutrient supply in just the first week of life is associated with better infant neurodevelopment after correcting for likely confounders; an extra 10 kcal/kg/day energy or an extra 1 g/kg/day protein was associated with a staggering 4.6- or 8.2-point higher developmental score using Bayley Scale of Infant Development (BSID) at 18 months age [16]. A large observational study in extremely preterm infants from Sweden (Express study) showed that energy intakes over the first 4 weeks of life were associated with retinopathy of prematurity (ROP): for every 10 kcal/kg/day increase in energy intakes, there was a 24% reduction in ROP after controlling for known confounders [17]. Whilst the risks for ROP are multifactorial, it is likely that the reduced risk of ROP was modulated in part via effects on IGF-1. An RCT providing higher nutrient intakes using both enteral nutrition and PN over the first few weeks of life resulted in greater weight gain, but most impressively resulted in measurable differences using MRI at term-corrected age in specific brain regions [18, 19]. This study showed that there was a larger Superior Longitudinal Fasciculus in those receiving enhanced intakes which is known to be involved in motor function, perception, and language. Finally, in long-term follow-up studies of studies initiated by Lucas' group [20], there were significant differences detected at 16 years of age. In this study, adolescents who had received higher nutrient intakes (compared to control) for only 4 weeks on average on the NICU, had verbal IQ that was 8 points higher, matched by MRI evidence of a larger-sized caudate nucleus. Although there are associations between weight gain in the postdischarge period and subsequent brain development, RCTs do not show a clear role for macronutrient enrichment of formula to improve brain outcomes at this stage, although further studies are needed [21, 22].

Numerous observational studies show strong associations between the amount of HM received as a preterm infant and later developmental and cognitive outcome, although there are, of course, no RCTs. Again, the studies of Lucas [23] provide the strongest evidence to show that the amount of HM received as a preterm infant affects verbal and full-scale IQ and white matter volume on

MRI conducted 15 years later. However, RCTs exploring the impact of DHM on later brain development do not show any consistent developmental advantage on BSID scores in infancy [24]. This might be because DHM contains relatively less macronutrients (and therefore needs greater fortification), or because the processing of DHM (collection, pasteurization, storage, transport etc.) affects key functional components that result in better brain outcomes. DHM might still be beneficial if it reduces the incidence of NEC [25] that damages the brain but will not result in the long-term brain advantages seen with MOM.

Micronutrients, Trace Elements, and the Brain

There are several micronutrients that are critical for brain development; however, there is relatively little evidence that providing intakes greater than currently recommended is beneficial. Iron is a critical nutrient for the developing brain, and suboptimal supply in 1–2 year-old infants results in worse BSID scores even in the absence of anemia [26]. However, most preterm infants will not become iron deficient if they receive recommended intakes (~2–3 mg/kg/day starting at around 3 weeks of age) whilst on the NICU and in the postdischarge period. Other metals such as zinc and selenium will also be essential, but again there is limited evidence of widespread deficiency when infants are fed recommended dietary intakes on the NICU. Iodine deficiency is a common cause of impaired brain development worldwide, although the incidence is much lower now that there is widespread use of iodinated salt. Many PN solutions appear to contain little or no iodine, and there was concern that this might be the cause of the commonly observed suboptimal thyroid function in preterm infants. However, a large RCT failed to show consistent benefits of iodine supplementation suggesting most infants somehow receive sufficient intakes, perhaps due to even very small amounts of contamination from iodine antisepsis in the mother or neonate, or some other route [27]. Whilst there is an understandable focus on nutrients that are well known to impact on brain development such as protein, energy, iron, fatty acids, etc., it is important to remember that no nutrients function in isolation, and humans require a diet that provides every essential nutrient for brain development to progress normally. Dietary nutrients may affect brain outcomes either by acting as substrate for new brain tissue, by providing energy to power the system, or by acting as cofactors, enzymes, or signaling compounds. Furthermore, there is strong evidence that certain nutrients such as DHA, folate, B_{12}, iron etc. are involved in several epigenetic processes that may also impact on brain development.

Supplemental Nutrients

There have been some interesting RCTs in recent years suggesting that specific components present in HM might improve brain outcomes. In term infants, milk fat globule membrane supplementation appears to improve brain outcomes in formula-fed infants [28], but no data exist in preterm infants. Sphingomyelin supplementation has been shown to possibly improve neurological outcomes in one very small study, but no confirmatory data exist [29]. The normal transplacental transfer of DHA to the developing fetus does not occur in preterm infants who might also have higher demands. Breastmilk concentrations of DHA also appear to be lower in mother's providing HM compared to several years ago, potentially reflecting differences in maternal dietary intakes. However, supplementing infants or their mothers with DHA is not straightforward, and RCTs have shown slightly higher rates of chronic lung disease in infants receiving higher intakes. This might be due to an imbalance that could be corrected by combined supplementation with arachidonic acid (AA). Indeed, a recent RCT in over 200 Swedish infants showed a 50% reduction in ROP in infants receiving both DHA and AA with no adverse impact on BPD rates [30]. Finally, there are basic scientific data to suggest that inadequate choline intakes might be more common than expected, and that these may adversely impact on brain development [31]. A small RCT in infants at high risk of cerebral palsy showed better language development using the BSID at 2 years of age when infants received a nutrient supplement containing DHA, choline, and a nucleotide [13]. Further large RCTs are being planned.

Conclusions

Preterm infants are at high risk of adverse brain outcomes that will have lifelong consequences on neurocognitive function. Damage to the brain may be a direct consequence of intraventricular hemorrhage or periventricular leukomalacia but might also be secondary to the cytokine storm seen in association with NEC or sepsis which damages white matter. Even in the absence of direct damage, the very high nutrient demands, and limited stores of preterm infants mean they are at high risk of malnutrition. This may limit brain growth as well as adversely affecting the time-dependent coordinated development of complex brain pathways that is especially active in early life. Careful attention to nutritional management in preterm infants has the potential to prevent damage by reducing the risk of NEC, and by ensuring adequate nutrients for brain tissue accretion and sufficient energy to "drive" the process. Whilst further studies are needed, there is also reason to hope that in the future, supplemental "functional" nutrients such as HMOs, DHA, choline, or other fatty acids and phospholipids may improve outcomes.

Conflict of Interest Statement

Dr. Embleton declares research funding to his organization from Danone Early Life Nutrition and Prolacta Bioscience US; lecture honoraria from Nestlé Nutrition Institute and Baxter. Dr. Granger and Dr. Chmelova declare no conflicts.

References

1 Embleton ND. Early nutrition and later outcomes in preterm infants. World Rev Nutr Diet. 2013;106:26–32.
2 Cleminson JS, Zalewski SP, Embleton ND. Nutrition in the preterm infant: what's new? Curr Opin Clin Nutr Metab Care. 2016;19(3):220–5.
3 Embleton NDE, Pang N, Cooke RJ, et al. Postnatal malnutrition and growth retardation: an inevitable consequence of current recommendations in preterm infants? Pediatrics. 2001;107:270–3.
4 Agostoni C, Buonocore G, Carnielli VP, et al. Enteral nutrient supply for preterm infants: commentary from the European Society of Paediatric Gastroenterology, Hepatology and Nutrition Committee on Nutrition. J Pediatr Gastroenterol. Nutr. 2010;50:85–91.
5 Granger CL, Embleton ND, Palmer JM, et al. Maternal Breast milk, infant gut microbiome, and the impact on preterm infant health. Acta Paediatr. 2021 Feb;110(2):450–457.
6 Masi A, Embleton N, Lamb C, et al. Human milk oligosaccharide DSLNT and gut microbiome in preterm infants predicts necrotising enterocolitis. Gut. 2020 Dec 16;gutjnl-2020-322771.
7 Williams T, Nair H, Simpson J, et al. Use of donor human milk and maternal breastfeeding rates: a systematic review. J Hum Lact. 2016;32:212–20.
8 Georgieff MK, Brunette KE, Tran PV. Early life nutrition and neural plasticity. Dev Psychopathol. 2015;27(2):411–23.
9 Wachs TD, Georgieff M, Cusick S, et al. Issues in the timing of integrated early interventions: contributions from nutrition, neuroscience, and psychological research. Ann NY Acad Sci. 2014;1308:89–106.
10 Hansen-Pupp I, Löfqvist C, Polberger S, et al. Influence of insulin-like growth factor I and nutrition during phases of postnatal growth in very preterm infants. Pediatr Res. 2011 May;69(5 Pt 1):448–53.
11 Roze JC, Darmaun D, Boquien CY, et al. The apparent breastfeeding paradox in very preterm infants: relationship between breast feeding, early weight gain and neurodevelopment based on results from two cohorts, EPIPAGE and LIFT. BMJ Open. 2012 Apr;2(2):e000834.
12 Dabydeen L, Thomas JE, Aston TJ, et al. High-energy and -protein diet increases brain and corticospinal tract growth in term and preterm infants after perinatal brain injury. Pediatrics. 2008;121:148–56.
13 Andrew MJ, Parr JR, Montague-Johnson C, et al. Neurodevelopmental outcome of nutritional intervention in newborn infants at risk of neurodevelopmental impairment: the Dolphin neonatal double-blind randomized controlled trial. Dev Med Child Neurol. 2018;60:906–13.
14 Roze E, Ta BDP, Van Der Ree MH, et al. Functional impairments at school age of children with necrotizing enterocolitis or spontaneous intestinal perforation. Pediatr Res. 2011;70:619–25.
15 Hackam DJ, Sodhi CP, Good M. New insights into necrotizing enterocolitis: from laboratory observation to personalized prevention and treatment. J Pediatr Surg. 2019 Mar;54(3):398–404.
16 Stephens BE, Walden RV, Gargus RA, et al. First-week protein and energy intakes are associated with 18-month developmental outcomes in extremely low birth weight infants. Paediatrics. 2009 May;123(5):1337–43.
17 Stoltz Sjostrom E, Lundgren P, Ohlund I, et al. Low energy intake during the first 4 weeks of life increases the risk for severe retinopathy of prematurity in extremely preterm infants. Arch Dis Child Fetal Neonatal Ed. 2016 Mar;101(2): F108–13.

18 Strommen K, Blakstad EW, Moltu SJ, et al. En-hanced nutrient supply to very low birth weight infants is associated with improved white matter maturation and head growth. Neonatology. 2015;107:68–75.

19 Strømmen K, Haag A, Moltu SJ, et al. Enhanced nutrient supply to very low birth weight infants is associated with higher blood amino acid concentrations and improved growth. Clin Nutr ESPEN. 2017;18:16–22.

20 Isaacs EB, Morley R, Lucas A. Early diet and general cognitive outcome at adolescence in children born at or below 30 weeks gestation. J Pediatr. 2009;155:229–34.

21 Embleton ND, Wood CL, Pearce MS, et al. Early diet in preterm infants and later cognition: 10-year follow-up of a randomized controlled trial. Pediatr Res. 2021 May;89(6):1442–1446.

22 Teller IC, Embleton ND, Griffin IJ, et al. Post-discharge formula feeding in preterm infants: a systematic review mapping evidence about the role of macronutrient enrichment. Clin Nutr. 2016 Aug;35(4):791–801.

23 Lucas A. Post-discharge nutrition and growth: relationship to later cognition. Pediatr Res. 2021;i:1–2.

24 O'Connor DL, Gibbins S, Kiss A, et al. Effect of supplemental donor human milk compared with preterm formula on neurodevelopment of very low-birth-weight infants at 18 months. JAMA. 2016;316:1897.

25 Quigley M, Embleton ND, McGuire W. Formula versus donor breast milk for feeding preterm or low birth weight infants. Cochrane Database Syst Rev. 2019 Jul 19;7(7):CD002971.

26 Lozoff B, Beard J, Connor J, et al. Long-lasting neural and behavioral effects of iron deficiency in infancy. Nutr Rev. 2006 May;64(5 Pt 2):S34–43; discussion S72–91.

27 Williams FLR, Ogston S, Hume R, et al. Supplemental iodide for preterm infants and developmental outcomes at 2 years: an RCT. Pediatrics. 2017 May;139(5):e20163703.

28 Timby N, Domellöf E, Hernell O, et al. Neurodevelopment, nutrition, and growth until 12 mo of age in infants fed a low-energy, low-protein formula supplemented with bovine milk fat globule membranes: a randomized controlled trial. Am J Clin Nutr. 2014;99:860–8.

29 Tanaka K, Hosozawa M, Kudo N, et al. The pilot study: Sphingomyelin-fortified milk has a positive association with the neurobehavioural development of very low birth weight infants during infancy, randomized control trial. Brain Dev. 2013;35:45–62.

30 Hellström A. Effect of enteral lipid supplement on severe retinopathy of prematurity: a randomized clinical trial. JAMA Pediatr. 2021 Apr;175(4):359–367.

31 Caudill MA, Strupp BJ, Muscalu L, et al. Maternal choline supplementation during the third trimester of pregnancy improves infant information processing speed: a randomized, double-blind, controlled feeding study. FASEB J. 2018;32:2172–80.

Nicholas D. Embleton
Newcastle Hospitals
NHS Foundation Trust
Newcastle University
Royal Victoria Infirmary
Newcastle upon Tyne NE1 4LP
UK
nicholas.embleton@ncl.ac.uk

Published online: May 10, 2022

Embleton ND, Haschke F, Bode L (eds): Strategies in Neonatal Care to Promote Optimized Growth and Development: Focus on Low Birth Weight Infants. 96th Nestlé Nutrition Institute Workshop, May 2021. Nestlé Nutr Inst Workshop Ser. Basel, Karger, 2022, vol 96, pp 34–44 (DOI: 10.1159/000519399)

Postdischarge Nutrition of Preterm Infants: Breastfeeding, Complementary Foods, Eating Behavior and Feeding Problems

Nadja Haiden

Departments of Pediatrics and Clinical Pharmacology, Medical University Vienna, Vienna, Austria

Abstract

In preterm infants, the key goals of nutrition are to establish adequate growth and to contribute to appropriate neurodevelopmental outcome. In this context, the postdischarge period is crucial to establish catch-up growth and avoid wrong metabolic programming caused by overfeeding. Breastfeeding is strongly recommended, and for preterm infants the European Society for Gastroenterology, Hepatology, and Nutrition (ESPGHAN) suggests fortifying breastmilk after discharge up to term in appropriate growing infants and up to 3 months in growth-retarded infants. If breastfeeding is not possible, postdischarge formula should be fed at least up to term. However, the effects of a higher nutrient density and energy administered by breastmilk fortification or postdischarge formula on growth and neurodevelopmental outcome are limited or missing but might have a positive impact on lung function and vision later in life. Moreover, little is known on the optimal timepoint to introduce solids in preterm infants. Data from observational studies have shown that preterm infants are weaned early in life around 13–15 weeks of corrected age. The degree of prematurity and use of formula are major determinants for early complementary feeding introduction. It is emphasized that there should be a strong focus on the infant's anatomical, physiological, and oral-motor readiness to receive foods other than breast milk or formula. Feeding problems and preterm's eating difficulties are common, and especially in the very immature population approximately 30% show oro-motor dysfunction or avoidant behavior at 3 months. An individualized approach according to the infant's neurological ability and nutritional status seems to be the best practice when introducing complementary feeding in preterm infants especially in the absence of evidence-based guidelines.

The optimal nutrition of preterm infants during their first weeks of life is a difficult task for neonatologists and remains a challenge even after discharge. As a consequence of prematurity, preterm infants have high needs for nutrients on the one hand and an organ immaturity on the other hand, which contributes to the difficulty of achieving dietary intakes that allow these infants to grow adequately.

They are also at high risk for delaying their neurodevelopmental milestones resulting in poor feeding skills and feeding problems. Overall, preterm infants may be sleepier at the time of discharge and may have more difficulties in latching, sucking, and swallowing than full-term infants [1]. Additionally, the preterm population is exceptionally inhomogeneous, primarily because of the variation in gestational age from 22 to 36 weeks but also due to the affection by persistent morbidities retarding normal growth (e.g., chronic lung disease, short bowel syndrome, etc.). These infants have higher nutritional requirements and/or the need to limit the volume of feeds consumed [2]. Finally, preterm infants tend to be discharged from the hospital earlier than the expected term. For the postdischarge period, it is important to define the nutritional requirements, to individualize the nutritional approach, and to consider feeding skills and emotional factors [2].

Optimal Growth after Discharge

In preterm infants, the key issue of perinatal and postdischarge nutrition is to establish adequate growth and appropriate neurodevelopmental outcome. A few years ago, the optimal growth trajectories of preterm infants during their early postnatal period were redefined: Rochow et al. [3] nicely showed that the "physiologic" growth trajectory of preterm infants is 1 SDS below their birth percentile. This is attributed to the fact that preterm infants have a higher body water content than term infants which results in a higher postnatal extracellular water loss [3]. A single chart cannot be used to monitor and plot the growth of infants during their initial hospital course and through the early discharge period, when the risk of growth restriction is greatest. To address this, a combination of the Fenton growth charts [4] and the WHO growth charts [5] is helpful (Fig. 1 [6]). The one-time postnatal contraction of extracellular water spaces occurs after preterm birth, leading to a temporary separation of growth curves by the equivalent of approximately −0.8 z-scores and re-emerging after 42 + 0/7 weeks (Fig. 1) [6].

But what is the optimal postdischarge growth velocity? ESPGHAN classified postdischarge growth into four distinct patterns [7]: (1) neonates adequate for

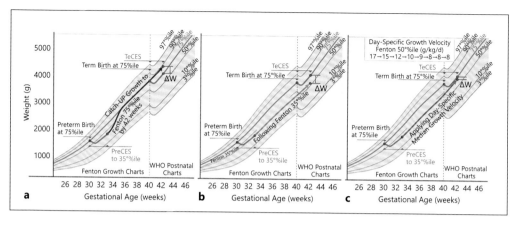

Fig. 1. Three examples for different postnatal growth trajectories of preterm infants [6]. **a** Birth-weight-percentile approach. After premature contraction of extracellular spaces (PreCES [blue]) and postnatal adaptation, infant catch-up growth (dark blue) to the percentile curve of the birth weight on Fenton chart until 42+0/7 weeks. **b** Postnatal-percentile approach. After PreCES, infants follow the percentile achieved (orange) on Fenton chart at day of life 21 until 42 + 0/7 weeks. **c** Fetal-median-growth and growth-velocity approach. Application of Fenton day-specific median growth velocities or day-specific median growth velocities adjusted by a factor from day of life 21 until 42 + 0/7 weeks (pink). ΔW indicates difference between target WHOGS weight at 42 + 0/7 weeks PMA and predicted individual growth trajectory weight using either postnatal-percentile approach, fetal-median-growth approach, or growth-velocity approach. PMA, postmenstrual age; TeCES, term contraction of extracellular spaces; WHOGS, World Health Organization growth standards. Reproduced from Landau-Crangle et al. [6] (Creative Commons Attribution-NonCommercial License).

gestational age (AGA) at birth without extrauterine growth retardation (EUGR); (2) neonates AGA at birth but with EUGR; (3) neonates small for gestational age (SGA) at birth without catch-up growth at discharge; (4) neonates SGA at birth but with early catch-up growth at discharge. ESPGHAN recommended that all preterm infants should receive either fortified breastmilk or a special postdischarge formula at least until a postconceptional age of 40 weeks. Infants discharged with a subnormal weight (<10th percentile) for postconceptional age and thus with an increased risk of long-term growth failure should receive fortified breastmilk or postdischarge formula possibly until about 52 weeks. These recommendations were published in 2006 and since then a lot of research on metabolic programming especially in SGA infants has been published which indicates that these recommendations should be updated. Postdischarge studies comparing enriched versus standard nutrition highlighted the ability of some preterm infants – like their term counterparts – to regulate their intake volume to compensate for differences in energy density between formulas [8]. This is only applicable to preterm babies reaching term due date and beyond as it has been reported that many less mature preterm babies are not able to compensate for low nutrient density feedings due to immature feeding skills [9]. Still, there is no doubt that infants with EUGR and a complicated neonatal course need enhanced nutrients for catch up growth.

Postdischarge Nutrition

From the nutritional aspect, the time after hospital discharge up to the end of the first year of life can be divided into 2 parts: the period of exclusive nursing or formula feeding and the period when complementary feeding is started in addition to breast- or formula feeding.

There is no doubt that breastmilk is the best source of nutrition for all infants but especially for those born preterm. So far, 3 randomized controlled trials are available investigating different methods of breastmilk fortification while exclusively breastfeeding after discharge and their effect on growth and neurodevelopmental outcome. In the largest study published by Zachariassen et al. [10], the entire dose of a commercial human milk fortifier (HMF) was added into one bottle of pumped breastmilk per day up to 4 months corrected age. No effect on growth was found at 3 or 12 months of age. However, a follow-up study of the cohort reported a better lung function at 6 years [11]. In a second study, HMF was administered by cup twice a day up to 12 weeks after discharge [12]. The intervention induced better weight, length, head growth, and bone mineral density in babies with birth weight <1,250 g which was persisting up to 1 year of age [13] as well as better visual function [14]. In the third study, preterm infants received HMF added to expressed breastmilk twice a day for 4–6 months of corrected age in otherwise to exclusive breastfeeding [15]. This study mainly focused on neurodevelopmental outcome at 12 months and did not provide anthropometric outcomes. None of the studies reported any adverse effects on breastfeeding behavior, but unfortunately there was no positive effect on neurodevelopmental outcome. However, there seems to be an association between exclusive breastfeeding at discharge and improved cognitive outcomes despite suboptimal initial weight gain [16]. Weight gain does not necessarily reflect body composition changes, which can be summarized as the "apparent breastfeeding paradox." That means that although breastfeeding can be associated with a significantly increased risk of losing one weight z-score during hospitalization, head circumference z-scores are higher than 0.5 at 2 years [17] and at 5 years [18] of age with a significantly decreased risk for suboptimal neurodevelopmental assessment [16].

If the mother is not able to breastfeed, ESPGHAN recommends to feed postdischarge formula up to at least 40 weeks, and in growth-retarded infants up to

52 weeks [19]. Postdischarge formula has a higher nutrient and energy density (74 kcal/100 mL) ranging between preterm and term formula. A meta-analysis addressed the question if feeding formulas enriched with energy, protein, and micronutrients to preterm infants after hospital discharge would result in catch-up growth [20]. Accelerated weight gain and crossing of body mass index percentiles might be associated with altered fat distribution and related "programmed" metabolic consequences that may increase the risk of insulin resistance and cardiovascular disease later in life [20]. However, because preterm infants fed in response to hunger and satiation cues (demand or responsive feeding) can adjust their volume of intake according to the energy density of formula, infants may consume less nutrient-enriched milk than standard formula [20]. Consequently, infants fed responsively with preterm or postdischarge formula may not receive more energy (or other nutrients) than infants fed standard term formula. The meta-analysis did not provide evidence that feeding postdischarge formula versus standard term formula (~67 kcal/100 mL) to preterm infants after hospital discharge affects growth parameters up to 12–18 months or neurodevelopmental outcome [20].

Although there are no effects of postdischarge formula on outcome with 1 year, there seems to be an association of early infant growth and later cognition. Data of a 10-year follow-up study showed that weight gain in the first 3 months was significantly associated with improved intelligence quotient and freedom from distractibility subsets of the Wechsler Intelligence Scale for children, which remained significant even after adjusting for weight gain [21]. These data are in line with other studies in preterm infants indicating that infants with a better weight gain between term and 4 months corrected age have a higher developmental score at 18 months [22] and another study showing that each unit increase in weight SDS between term and 1 year of age was associated with a 1.9-point IQ advantage at 8 years of age [23]. Therefore, it is likely that the 3–4 months after term remain a potentially important period for optimizing brain development through dietary management.

Complementary Feeding in Preterm Infants

In full-term infants, ESPGHAN [24, 25] recommends a stepwise introduction of complementary food (CF) between the 17th and 26th week of life. In preterm infants, guidelines on the optimal time for starting solids and the ideal composition of CF meeting their special requirements are missing [26, 27]. Observational studies have shown that in general solids are introduced early to preterm infants [28–30]. An Italian study documented that infants born between 24 and 32 weeks were weaned from exclusive nursing or formula feeding at 13 weeks corrected for term, while more mature infants born between 33 and 36 weeks were weaned at 15 weeks corrected for term [26] indicating that the degree of prematurity is a major determinant for CF introduction. The odds for being weaned before 4 months are 9.9 times higher in infants born between 22 and 32 weeks' gestation, and 6.19 higher in infants born between 33 and 36 weeks' gestation when compared with term infants [31]. Another interesting issue was that in general formula-fed infants are weaned earlier than breastfed infants or infants on mixed feeding [26].

To date, only 2 RCTs have investigated time of introduction and nutritional quality of solids for preterm infants. A study which was published before postdischarge fortification of breastmilk and postdischarge formula were introduced randomized preterm infants either into a "preterm weaning strategy (PWS)" group or to a control group [32]. Infants in the PWS group received high-energy, high-protein, semisolid foods together with a preterm infant formula starting at 13 weeks of uncorrected age, provided they had reached at least 3.5 kg body weight. Infants in the control group were started on CF at 17 weeks of uncorrected age, provided they weighed at least 5 kg, and no specific advice for food quality was given. At 12 months of age, infants in the PWS group had greater length compared to those in the control group, with no differences in weight or head circumference [32]. A more recent RCT from India published in 2017 could not find an effect of CF introduction at 4 versus 6 months on weight for age z-scores, other anthropometric parameters, or neurodevelopmental outcome at 1 year in preterm infants with a GA <34 weeks [33]. Breastfeeding, type of formula or maternal education did not influence results. However, this study was conducted in a lower/middle-income country indicating that setting and results cannot be transferred to high-income countries. In this study, infants in both groups showed a remarkable loss in z-scores of –2.8 around term, which does not correspond to normal growth trajectories in European cohorts [34]. This growth retardation persisted up to 1 year of corrected age, where z-score loss was still –1.6 in both groups (Fig. 2). The results of the study also highlight the importance of quality of solid foods indicating that a nutrient-rich diet is important in these infants. Also, little is known about the timing of introduction of single food groups in preterm infants. In an internet survey among Italian pediatricians, Baldassarre et al. [35] investigated: (1) timing of the introduction of CFs to preterm newborns; (2) type of CFs introduced; (3) vitamin D and iron supplementations. Results showed that the decision to introduce solids was mainly based on the infants' age (44%). 58% of the pediatricians recommended to start at corrected age (mean 5.5 months), and 42% recommended to start at the chronological age (mean 5.6 months), indicating that there is no consensus concerning chronological or corrected age. Only 18% of the pediatricians con-

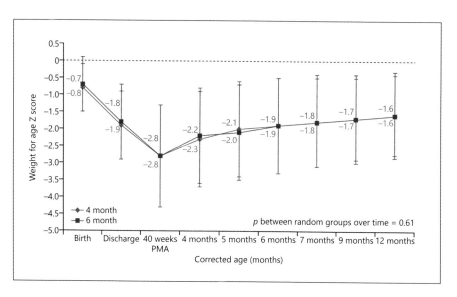

Fig. 2. Change in weight for age z-scores among study infants over the time per study group [32]. Blue symbols and lines, complementary food was introduced at 4 months' PMA; red symbols and lines, complementary food was introduced at 6 months' PMA. Includes data only for infants who completed 12-month follow-up. Data are in mean (SD). PMA, postmenstrual age [32].

sidered the neurological ability of the infants to accept solids, which is especially important in extremely immature infants. Parents started with fruits, vegetables, oil, and cereals at 5.5 months, followed by meat (5.6 months), gluten (5.8 months) milk products (7 months), fish (7.4 months), and egg (8.7 months) [35]. Approximately 90% of the infants received iron supplements up to 9.3 months, which is important, as preterm infants often have depleted iron stores and require extra iron intake during their first year of life. Vitamin D was provided up to 21.1 months [35]. The introduction of single food groups was strongly affected by local availability of aliments as well as cultural habits and practices. Data from high-quality, prospective randomized trials investigating the optimal timepoint for CF introduction under consideration of chronological or corrected age, the optimal composition, and appropriate supplements such as vitamin D or iron are not available so far.

Neurological Ability and Introduction of CF

The key issue for the introduction of CFs is the infant's anatomical, physiological, and oral-motor readiness to receive foods other than breast milk or formula.

Once an infant has developed an apparent interest in non-milk foods and feeding, the changes that are required for progressing from a liquid to a semi-solid and solid diet are [36]:

1. Anatomical changes in the oral cavity
2. The disappearance or diminishing of reflexes present at birth that coordinate suckling, swallowing and respiration, and protect the infant from aspiration and choking (i.e., the extrusion reflex of the tongue), in favor of more voluntary movements, and
3. The development of gross motor skills (head and trunk control to allow an improved movement of the jaw) and fine motor skills (lip, tongue, and jaw movements).

The age range at which preterm infants attain these developmental milestones are related to their immaturity, morbidities, and their perinatal course. Furthermore, feeding problems and preterm's eating difficulties are also related to psychological roots caused by the multiple and unpleasant procedures undergone during hospitalization (e.g., tube feeding, intubation, etc.) [2]. In term infants, the earliest gross motor skills indicative of developmental readiness for spoon-feeding of pureed foods (i.e., holding the head in midline when in supine position and to control its head well when pulled to sitting or at aided sitting) can be observed between 3 and 4 months of age [36]. At this age, it can be assumed that the rooting and the extrusion reflexes may have also diminished in some infants. The gross motor skill indicative of developmental readiness for self-feeding finger foods (i.e., sitting without support) can be observed in some infants at 4 months, but more commonly between 5 and 7 months of age. In preterm infants, the necessary developmental milestones for feeding are also reached around the same age range (post-term), depending on the severity of illness experienced during the neonatal period, the degree of prematurity, and any sequelae [36].

A large prospective study in early (GA <34 weeks; $n = 319$) and late (GA 34–37 weeks; $n = 571$) preterm infants investigated the incidence of postdischarge feeding dysfunction and hospital/subspecialty visits for feeding problems during the first year of life [37]. Twenty-nine and 17% of the early preterm and late preterm infants showed oro-motoric dysfunction, respectively. Corresponding percentages for avoidant behavior at 3 months were 33 and 29% [37]. Formula feeding increases the chance of presenting complementary feeding difficulties by 41% (OR; 0.27–7.13) when compared to exclusive breastfeeding and mixed feeding [38]. In most of the infants, the symptoms disappeared during the first year of life, but these results highlight that pediatricians should screen preterm infants for feeding dysfunction during their first year of life [37]. Preterm infants who show oral dysfunctions need a multidisciplinary follow-up that must include a nutritionist and a speech therapist specializing in oral function [2].

An individualized approach according to the infant's neurological ability and nutritional status seems to be the best practice when introducing complementary feeding in preterm infants especially in the absence of evidence-based guidelines.

Conclusion

Preterm infants with EUGR and a complicated neonatal course need food with a higher nutritional density to establish postnatal catch-up growth and proper development. So far, it is not clear what the optimal growth velocity is to guarantee an optimal neurodevelopmental outcome and appropriate metabolic programming in the period after discharge from hospital, during their first year, and later in life. Fortification of breastmilk after discharge might be an opportunity to improve growth, but studies have shown conflicting results. If breastfeeding is not possible, postdischarge formulas are available but do not affect postnatal growth. The available evidence suggests that there is no specific timing for the introduction of solids. This issue needs more research from high-quality RCTs. Complementary feeding should be introduced following an individualized evaluation which is based on infants' development rather than corrected or postnatal age. Furthermore, preterm infants who have developed oral dysfunction need support by a multidisciplinary team that must include pediatricians, nutritionists, and speech therapists specialized in oral function.

Conflict of Interest Statement

N.H. receives honoraria for lectures from Nestlé, Baxter, Danone, Novalac, and MUM. The author has no other conflicts of interest to declare.

References

1 Lapillonne A. Feeding the preterm infant after discharge. World Rev Nutr Diet. 2014;110:264–77.
2 Crippa BL, Morniroli D, Baldassarre ME, et al. Preterm's nutrition from hospital to solid foods: are we still navigating by sight? Nutrients. 2020 Nov;12(12).
3 Rochow N, Raja P, Liu K, et al. Physiological adjustment to postnatal growth trajectories in healthy preterm infants. Pediatr Res. 2016 06;79(6):870–9.
4 Fenton TR, Kim JH. A systematic review and meta-analysis to revise the Fenton growth chart for preterm infants. BMC Pediatr. 2013 Apr;13:59.
5 WHO Multicentre Growth Reference Study Group. WHO Child Growth Standards based on length/height, weight and age. Acta Paediatr Suppl. 2006 Apr;450:76–85.
6 Landau-Crangle E, Rochow N, Fenton TR, et al. Individualized postnatal growth trajectories for preterm infants. J Parenter Enteral Nutr. 2018 Aug;42(6):1084–92.

7   Aggett PJ, Agostoni C, Axelsson I, et al. Feeding preterm infants after hospital discharge: a commentary by the ESPGHAN Committee on Nutrition. J Pediatr Gastroenterol Nutr. 2006 May;42(5):596–603.

8   Arslanoglu S, Boquien CY, King C, et al. Fortification of human milk for preterm infants: update and recommendations of the European Milk Bank Association (EMBA) Working Group on Human Milk Fortification. Front Pediatr. 2019;7:76.

9   Arslanoglu S, Moro GE, Ziegler EE; The Wapm Working Group on Nutrition. Optimization of human milk fortification for preterm infants: new concepts and recommendations. J Perinat Med. 2010 May;38(3):233–8.

10 Zachariassen G, Faerk J, Grytter C, Esberg BH, Hjelmborg J, Mortensen S, et al. Nutrient enrichment of mother's milk and growth of very preterm infants after hospital discharge. Pediatrics. 2011 Apr;127(4):e995–e1003.

11 Toftlund LH, Agertoft L, Halken S, Zachariassen G. Improved lung function at age 6 in children born very preterm and fed extra protein post-discharge. Pediatr Allergy Immunol. 2019 02;30(1):47–54.

12 O'Connor DL, Khan S, Weishuhn K, et al. Growth and nutrient intakes of human milk-fed preterm infants provided with extra energy and nutrients after hospital discharge. Pediatrics. 2008 Apr;121(4):766–76.

13 Aimone A, Rovet J, Ward W, et al. Growth and body composition of human milk-fed premature infants provided with extra energy and nutrients early after hospital discharge: 1-year follow-up. J Pediatr Gastroenterol Nutr. 2009 Oct;49(4):456–66.

14 O'Connor DL, Weishuhn K, Rovet J, et al. Visual development of human milk-fed preterm infants provided with extra energy and nutrients after hospital discharge. JPEN J Parenter Enteral Nutr. 2012 May;36(3):349–53.

15 da Cunha RD, Lamy Filho F, Rafael EV, et al. Breast milk supplementation and preterm infant development after hospital discharge: a randomized clinical trial. J Pediatr (Rio J). 2016 Mar–Apr;92(2):136–42.

16 Rozé JC, Darmaun D, Boquien CY, et al. The apparent breastfeeding paradox in very preterm infants: relationship between breast feeding, early weight gain and neurodevelopment based on results from two cohorts, EPIPAGE and LIFT. BMJ Open. 2012;2(2):e000834.

17 Fewtrell MS, Morgan JB, Duggan C, et al. Optimal duration of exclusive breastfeeding: what is the evidence to support current recommendations? Am J Clin Nutr. 2007 Feb;85(2):635S–38S.

18 Rozé JC, Bureau-Rouger V, Beucher A, et al. [Follow-up network for newborns at risk for handicap in a French region]. Arch Pediatr. 2007 Sep;14(Suppl 1):S65–S70.

19 Agostoni C, Buonocore G, Carnielli VP, et al. Enteral nutrient supply for preterm infants: commentary from the European Society of Paediatric Gastroenterology, Hepatology and Nutrition Committee on Nutrition. J Pediatr Gastroenterol Nutr. 2010;50(1):85–91.

20 Young L, Embleton ND, McGuire W. Nutrient-enriched formula versus standard formula for preterm infants following hospital discharge. Cochrane Database Syst Rev. 2016 12;12:CD004696.

21 Embleton ND, Wood CL, Pearce MS, et al. Early diet in preterm infants and later cognition: 10-year follow-up of a randomized controlled trial. Pediatr Res. 2021 May;89(6):1442–46.

22 Belfort MB, Ehrenkranz RA. Neurodevelopmental outcomes and nutritional strategies in very low birth weight infants. Semin Fetal Neonatal Med. 2017;22(1):42–48.

23 Belfort MB, Martin CR, Smith VC, et al. Infant weight gain and school-age blood pressure and cognition in former preterm infants. Pediatrics. 2010 Jun;125(6):e1419–e26.

24 Agostoni C, Decsi T, Fewtrell M, et al. Complementary feeding: a commentary by the ESPGHAN Committee on Nutrition. J Pediatr Gastroenterol Nutr. 2008 Jan;46(1):99–110.

25 Fewtrell M, Bronsky J, Campoy C, et al. Complementary Feeding: A Position Paper by the European Society for Paediatric Gastroenterology, Hepatology, and Nutrition (ESPGHAN) Committee on Nutrition. J Pediatr Gastroenterol Nutr. 2017 01;64(1):119–32.

26 Fanaro S, Borsari G, Vigi V. Complementary feeding practices in preterm infants: an observational study in a cohort of Italian infants. J Pediatr Gastroenterol Nutr. 2007 Dec;45(Suppl 3):S210–S4.

27 Fanaro S, Vigi V. Weaning preterm infants: an open issue. J Pediatr Gastroenterol Nutr. 2007 Dec;45(Suppl 3):S204–S9.

28 Norris FJ, Larkin MS, Williams CM, et al. Factors affecting the introduction of complementary foods in the preterm infant. Eur J Clin Nutr. 2002 May;56(5):448–54.

29 Morgan JB, Williams P, Foote KD, Marriott LD. Do mothers understand healthy eating principles for low-birth-weight infants? Public Health Nutr. 2006 Sep;9(6):700–6.

30 Cleary J, Dalton SM, Harman A, Wright IM. Current practice in the introduction of solid foods for preterm infants. Public Health Nutr. 2020 01;23(1):94–101.

31 Braid S, Harvey EM, Bernstein J, Matoba N. Early introduction of complementary foods in preterm infants. J Pediatr Gastroenterol Nutr. 2015 Jun;60(6):811–8.

32 Marriott LD, Foote KD, Bishop JA, et al. Weaning preterm infants: a randomised controlled trial. Arch Dis Child Fetal Neonatal Ed. 2003 Jul;88(4):F302–F7.

33 Gupta S, Agarwal R, Aggarwal KC, et al. Complementary feeding at 4 versus 6 months of age for preterm infants born at less than 34 weeks of gestation: a randomised, open-label, multicentre trial. Lancet Glob Health. 2017;5(5):e501–e11.

34 El Rafei R, Jarreau PH, Norman M, et al. Variation in very preterm extrauterine growth in a European multicountry cohort. Arch Dis Child Fetal Neonatal Ed. 2021 May;106(3):316–23.

35 Baldassarre ME, Di Mauro A, Pedico A, et al. Weaning time in preterm infants: an audit of Italian Primary Care Paediatricians. Nutrients. 2018 May;10(5):616.

36 Castenmiller J, de Henauw S, Hirsch-Ernst KI, et al. Appropriate age range for introduction of complementary feeding into an infant's diet. EFSA J. 2019 Sep;17(9):e05780.

37 DeMauro SB, Patel PR, Medoff-Cooper B, et al. Postdischarge feeding patterns in early- and late-preterm infants. Clin Pediatr (Phila). 2011 Oct;50(10):957–62.

38 Menezes LVP, Steinberg C, Nóbrega AC. Complementary feeding in infants born prematurely. Codas. 2018 Oct;30(6):e20170157.

Nadja Haiden
Medical University of Vienna
Department of Clinical Pharmacology
Währinger Gürtel 18–20, AT–1090 Vienna
Austria
nadja.haiden@meduniwien.ac.at

Published online: May 10, 2022

Embleton ND, Haschke F, Bode L (eds): Strategies in Neonatal Care to Promote Optimized Growth and Development: Focus on Low Birth Weight Infants. 96th Nestlé Nutrition Institute Workshop, May 2021. Nestlé Nutr Inst Workshop Ser. Basel, Karger, 2022, vol 96, pp 45–53 (DOI: 10.1159/000519395)

Quality of Growth, Body Composition and Longer-Term Metabolic Outcomes

Neena Modi

Imperial College London, Chelsea and Westminster Hospital, London, UK

Abstract

The optimum growth and body composition of the preterm baby is unknown despite non-evidence-based opinions that this should mimic that of the full-term infant. The relationship between body composition at birth, in both preterm and full-term babies, and later cardio-metabolic outcomes is also unknown. Newborn body composition is influenced by maternal adiposity and diabetes, gestational age at birth, infant sex, and intrauterine growth restriction. Nutritional intake, breast and formula feeding, illness severity, and possibly growth velocity, are subsequent influences. It is not known whether differences in newborn body composition between ethnic groups are a consequence of genetic endowment, or intrauterine influences. Progress in this area requires funders and investigators to collaborate to establish high-quality, longitudinal cohort studies designed to have the ability to elicit causal inferences, and randomized controlled trials aiming to influence body composition that are of sufficient size to identify effects on functional outcomes at multiple time points across the life course, be generalizable across populations, and have power to detect important interactions.

Introduction

In children and adults, higher body mass index is associated with higher risk of cardiovascular morbidity and mortality. However, risk prediction in these populations is by no means precise, especially within the "normal" body mass index range, and if physical activity is not taken into account. This realization led to consideration of body composition, adipose tissue compartments and their distribution, and the ratio of adipose to lean body mass as biomarkers of risk. In infancy, the recognition that weight gain alone provides poor information about the accrual of adipose tissue and lean body mass has led to interest in body composition to guide nutritional practice. In addition, the American Academy of Pediatrics has recommended for many decades that it is desirable for the preterm infant to achieve the body composition and size of the baby born at full-term. However, although this recommendation has been repeated by many authors, whether or not this goal leads to improved long-term outcomes is unknown. Here, I will summarize knowledge of body composition in infancy, the determinants, and what is known about the relationship with functional health outcomes. I will avoid the term "low birth weight" as this is imprecise, failing to distinguish between low birth weight because of prematurity, and low birth weight because of growth restriction.

Assessing Body Composition in Infancy

A number of methods have been used to evaluate body composition in infants. These include indirect methods reliant on assumptions that vary in the strength of their applicability in infancy. These are isotope dilution studies, bioelectrical impedance, total electrical conductivity, dual-energy X-ray absorptiometry (DEXA), skinfold thickness measurements, and air displacement plethysmography. Adipose tissue magnetic resonance (MR) imaging is a direct, non-invasive method. Unlike DEXA, MR imaging is radiation-free and also enables quantification of regional adipose tissue depots, by taking serial "slice" images of the whole body, quantifying adipose and non-adipose compartments and summating them to provide an objective measure of each compartment (Fig. 1) [1]. However, infants must be still during whole-body MR imaging to avoid movement artefacts. As it would not be ethical to sedate infants for research MR imaging, the utility of this technique in infancy is limited to the early months when it is possible to use the "feed, swaddle, and sleep" technique [2].

The various methods of body composition analyses are not readily interchangeable, and the applicability of techniques changes with age, making longitudinal comparisons problematic. A further difficulty in combining or compar-

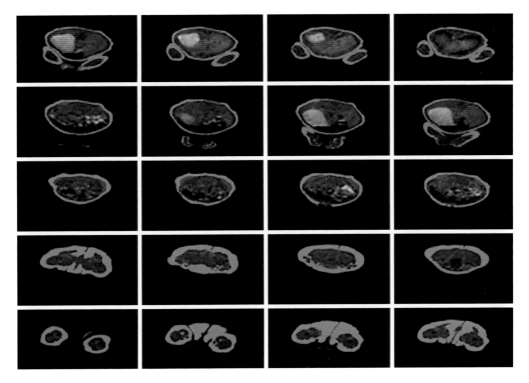

Fig. 1. Color-coded sequential images obtained during whole-body magnetic resonance imaging in a neonate; blue, deep subcutaneous and internal adipose tissue; green, superficial subcutaneous adipose tissue.

ing studies is the use of the terms "adipose tissue" and "fat" interchangeably. Adipose tissue consists of cellular membranes, predominantly protein and water, and intracellular lipid, which can be highly variable ranging, e.g. from 40% to over 90% in very obese individuals. As many authors do not provide clear definitions, it is often uncertain whether their data refer to adipose tissue, or lipid content. A further area of confusion is in the methods used to adjust adiposity for body size. This is important if comparisons in infants over time or between infants of different sizes are to be meaningful and reliably identify differences in relative adiposity. In infancy, presenting adipose tissue content as a percentage of body weight or a ratio to length is statistically unwise as the index is correlated with the denominator to a degree that changes over time. This is particularly problematic when comparing groups that differ in size, such as preterm and full-term infants. We examined the statistical validity of approaches used and recommend that in the neonatal period, adjustment of adipose tissue content is made using the denominator length^3 and in later infancy, length^2 [3].

Body Composition in the Neonatal Period and Infancy

Approximately 90% of third-trimester weight gain is adipose tissue, and human infants are among the most adipose of all species. Fat mass comprises around 10–15% of body weight in full-term human infants, though the range is wide, compared to about 3% in our closest primate relation, the chimpanzee. It is suggested that this substantial accrual of adipose tissue provides nutritional insurance, providing protection for the high energy requirement of the brain [4]. Human full-term infants experience a period of relative mandatory fasting immediately after birth, while maternal lactation is established and as colostrum is low in energy content. Thus, high adiposity of the human infant is normal and is amplified over the first 3–6 months [5, 6]. In contrast, very and extremely preterm infants miss out on third-trimester intrauterine development and are born with very little adipose tissue. This is also the case for babies who suffer intrauterine growth restriction; here, nutrition is directed towards the brain, leading to the phenomenon of "brain-sparing" and "asymmetrical growth restriction" where brain growth is sustained at the cost of somatic growth.

A number of factors influence body composition in infancy in addition to infant sex. Babies with intrauterine growth restriction have reduced adiposity. We compared adipose tissue content and distribution using MR imaging at birth and 6 weeks of age in appropriately grown and growth-restricted full-term infants [7]. At birth, adiposity was significantly less in growth-restricted infants, but by 6 weeks, they had shown complete catch-up in head growth and adiposity, but not length and weight. The highest adiposity at 6 weeks was seen in exclusively breastfed growth-restricted infant. There were no significant differences between the groups in adipose tissue distribution. We speculated as to whether adipose tissue quantity at birth is involved in the signaling of growth, especially catch-up head growth.

Maternal Phenotype

Maternal adiposity influences newborn body composition. We have shown that newborn adiposity and hepatic lipid increase across the normal range of maternal body mass index [8]. Newborn adiposity is increased in diabetic mothers [9] and amplified in early infancy even when hyperglycemia is well controlled and predominant breastfeeding [10]. As the risk of offspring developing diabetes is increased as much as 11-fold in diabetic and obese pregnancies, data such as these indicate that these may be the initiating determinants of a lifelong trajectory leading to adverse metabolic health, marked by aberrant neonatal body composition.

We studied whole-body adipose tissue content and partitioning in healthy full-term Asian Indian and white European newborn infants born in Pune, India, and London, UK, respectively [11]. The Indian babies were lighter and smaller and had similar whole-body adipose tissue content, but the distribution differed. The Indian babies had significantly greater absolute adiposity in all abdominal compartments (internal, deep subcutaneous, and superficial subcutaneous) and significantly less in the non-abdominal subcutaneous compartment. This led us to speculate that genetic determinants related to ethnicity, or intrauterine influences may contribute to higher cardiometabolic risk and marked predisposition to abdominal adiposity that is well-recognized in Indians and other south Asians. Of note, hyperinsulinemia appears to be present at birth in Indian babies [12]. Other authors have noted increased deep subcutaneous abdominal adipose tissue in Indian and Malay neonates in comparison with Indian infants [13]. Data such as these suggest that differences in body composition, in keeping with known ethnicity-related cardiometabolic disease susceptibility, are evident at birth. However, what is unknown is whether these indicate genetic differences in susceptibility, or the influence of the intrauterine environment, the extent to which differences persist as the children grow older and hence their predictive value to ethnic disparities in cardiometabolic disease in adult life.

Preterm Birth

By term, babies born preterm are significantly lighter and shorter than full-term infants. However, in our initial study comparing preterm-at-term and full-term infants, we found no significant differences in head circumference z-score or total adiposity, but a marked difference in adipose tissue distribution with a decrease in subcutaneous adipose tissue and increase in intra-abdominal adipose tissue in the former group [14]. We also showed that accelerated postnatal weight gain was accompanied by an increase in total and subcutaneous adiposity, and that the degree of illness severity while in the neonatal unit was associated with greater intra-abdominal adiposity.

Cerasani et al. [15] performed a literature review on human milk feeding, and growth and body composition in preterm infants. Their general conclusions are that most studies report that human milk feeding in preterm infants is positively associated with fat-free mass. The exception was our prespecified secondary analysis of pooled data from a randomized controlled trial in very preterm infants in which we found a predominant diet of formula compared with exclusive human milk was associated with higher lean body mass and weight, but not with greater adiposity at term age [16]. Cerasani et al. [15] also conclude that growth following hospital discharge does not appear to be associated with increased fat mass in exclusively human milk-fed preterm infants. We compared weight at term in preterm infants following surgically and medically managed necrotizing enterocolitis, in comparison to preterm infants that did not develop the disease [17]. We found that lower weight in the necrotizing enterocolitis group was due to a reduction in adipose tissue content but not lean body mass, leading us to suggest that typical preterm nutritional regimens may be inadequate to support rapid third-trimester deposition of adipose tissue. Similar findings of low fat-free mass at term in preterm compared with full-term babies have been found in a review of fat and fat-free mass from birth to 6 months [18]. Caution is advised in interpreting these studies because of variation in techniques, analytical methods, study design, and populations, and in particular as none have elucidated the relationship between body composition in infancy and later functional health outcomes.

Long-Term Metabolic Outcomes after Preterm Birth

A substantial and growing body of literature from around the world indicates that preterm birth is a risk factor for the early onset of diseases that are characteristic of ageing such hypertension, cardiovascular diseases, renal impairment, and diabetes, and are associated with altered body composition, especially intra-abdominal (visceral) adiposity [19]. Life span is also reduced following preterm birth [20]. Large-scale studies and meta-analyses [21, 22] have shown that adults born preterm have higher blood pressure and risk of hypertension than their full-term counterparts with average increases of around 4.2 mm Hg for systolic and 2.6 mm Hg for diastolic pressure [22]. Though often viewed as small at an individual level, these differences equate to important risks at a population level as a 2 mm Hg increase in diastolic pressure equates to a 10% increase in mortality from ischemic heart disease and stroke [23]. There also appears to be a clear correlation between higher systolic blood pressure and increasing immaturity, and raised systolic and diastolic blood pressures have been detected in preterm born children as young as 2–3 years old. Preterm birth increases the odds of developing the metabolic syndrome (insulin resistance, dyslipidemia, central obesity, and hypertension) with alterations in atherogenic biomarkers indicative of risk to future cardiovascular health, including total cholesterol, apoprotein B and lower high-density lipoprotein cholesterol, and in insulin resistance and sensitivity, detectable in infancy [19]. Preterm-born individuals are also at significantly increased risk of type 1 and type 2 diabetes [24]. We have shown that outwardly healthy young adults born preterm have altered body composition in comparison with full-term counterparts, marked by increases in intra-abdominal adiposity [25, 26]. Observations such as these have added to consideration of the possibility that body composition can be used to define risk, and responses to interventions, and to whether nutritional and other care practices in infancy might exacerbate these risks.

Evidence Gaps and Future Directions

Published literature to date is strong on associations but weak on the well-powered, longitudinal studies that are necessary to determine the predictive ability of body composition indices at a particular point in infancy, for later outcomes. The European Childhood Obesity Trial provides high-quality evidence in healthy, full-term babies, that protein intake in infancy is a causal determinant of later risk of obesity, abdominal adiposity, and renal function [27]. Equivalent data in growth-restricted and preterm infants is lacking [28]. The consequences of these knowledge gaps are that there is little to guide clinical nutritional practice. This leads on the one hand to wide variation in practice and on the other to didactic "expert" opinion-based guidelines. Both approaches engender anxiety among parents and clinicians and are dangerous for patients [28].

Descriptive studies are emerging that provide valuable reference data for investigators. A few birth cohort studies, such as Growing up in Singapore [13] and the Pune Maternal Nutrition Study [12] are evaluating the early developmental origins of cardiometabolic disease. The Guangzhou Preterm Birth Cohort Study [29] will carry out body composition assessment using DEXA at ages 3, 6, 12, and 18 years in preterm children. A search of birth cohorts (www.birthcohorts.net) on June 5th 2021 revealed no other preterm studies. Data are beginning to emerge that depict longitudinal changes in body composition [30]. However, what is urgently needed is for funders and investigators to collaborate to establish high-quality, longitudinal cohort studies designed to have ability to elicit causal inferences, and randomized controlled trials of sufficient size to identify relationships with functional outcomes at multiple time points across the life course, be generalizable across populations, and have power to detect important interactions.

Conflict of Interests Statement

The author reports grants outside the submitted work from the Medical Research Council, National Institute of Health Research, March of Dimes, British Heart Foundation, HCA International, Health Data Research UK, Shire Pharmaceuticals, Chiesi Pharmaceuticals, Prolacta Life Sciences, and Westminster Children's Research Fund; N.M. is a member of the Nestlé Scientific Advisory Board and accepts no personal remuneration for this role. N.M. reports travel and accommodation reimbursements from Chiesi, Nestlé, and Shire.

References

1 Harrington TAM, Thomas EL, Modi N, Frost G, Coutts GA, Bell JD. Fast and reproducible method for the direct quantitation of adipose tissue in newborn infants. Lipids. 2002;37:95–100.

2 Gale C, Jeffries S, Logan KM, et al. Avoiding sedation in research magnetic resonance imaging and spectroscopy in infants: our approach, success rate and prevalence of incidental findings. Arch Dis Child Fetal Neonatal Ed. 2013;98:F267–8.

3 Gale C, Santhakumaran S, Wells JCK, Modi N. Adjustment of directly measured adipose tissue volume in infants. Int J Obes (Lond) 2014;38:995–9.

4 Cunnane SC, Crawford MA. Survival of the fattest: fat babies were the key to evolution of the large human brain. Comp Biochem Physiol A Mol Integr Physiol. 2003;136:17–26.

5 Gale C, Logan KM, Santhakumaran S, et al. Effect of breastfeeding compared with formula feeding on infant body composition: a systematic review and meta-analysis. Am J Clin Nutr. 2012;95:656–69.

6 Gale C, Thomas EL, Jeffries S, et al. Adiposity and hepatic lipid in healthy full-term, breastfed, and formula-fed human infants: a prospective short-term longitudinal cohort study. Am J Clin Nutr. 2014;99:1034–40.

7 Modi N, Thomas EL, Harrington TAM, et al. Determinants of adiposity during preweaning postnatal growth in appropriately grown and growth-restricted term infants. Pediatr Res. 2006;60:345–8.

8 Modi N, Murgasova D, Ruager-Martin R, et al. The influence of maternal body mass index on infant adiposity and hepatic lipid content. Pediatr Res. 2011;70:287–91.

9 Logan KM, Gale C, Hyde MJ, Santhakumaran S, Modi N. Diabetes in pregnancy and infant adiposity: systematic review and meta-analysis. Arch Dis Child Fetal Neonatal Ed. 2017;102:F65–F72.

10 Logan KM, Emsley RJ, Jeffries S, et al. Development of early adiposity in infants of mothers with gestational diabetes mellitus. Diabetes Care. 2016;39:1045–51.

11 Modi N, Thomas EL, Uthaya S, et al. Whole body magnetic resonance imaging of healthy newborn infants demonstrates increased central adiposity in Asian Indians. Pediatr Res. 2009;65:584–587.

12 Yajnik CS, Lubree HG, Rege SS, et al. Adiposity and hyperinsulinemia in Indians are present at birth. J Clin Endocrinol Metab. 2002;87:5575–80.

13 Tint MT, Fortier MV, Godfrey KM, et al. Abdominal adipose tissue compartments vary with ethnicity in Asian neonates: Growing Up in Singapore Toward Healthy Outcomes birth cohort study. Am J Clin Nutr. 2016;103:1311–7.

14 Uthaya S, Thomas EL, Hamilton G, Bell J, Modi N. Altered adiposity after extremely preterm birth. Pediatr Res. 2005;57:211–5.

15 Cerasani J, Ceroni F, De Cosmi V, et al. Human milk feeding and preterm infants' growth and body composition: a literature review. Nutrients. 2020 Apr;12(4):1155.

16 Li Y, Liu X, Modi N, Uthaya S. Impact of breast milk intake on body composition at term in very preterm babies: secondary analysis of the Nutritional Evaluation and Optimisation in Neonates randomised controlled trial. Arch Dis Child Fetal Neonatal Ed. 2019;104:F306–12.

17 Binder C, Longford N, Gale C, Modi N, Uthaya S. Body composition following necrotising enterocolitis in preterm infants. Neonatology. 2018;113:242–8.

18 Hamatschek C, Yousuf EI, Möllers LS, et al. Fat and fat-free mass of preterm and term infants from birth to six months: a review of current evidence. Nutrients. 2020;12:288.

19 Prior E, Modi N. Adult outcomes after preterm birth. Postgrad Med J. 2020;96:619–22.

20 Crump C, Sundquist J, Winkleby MA, Sundquist K. Gestational age at birth and mortality from infancy into mid-adulthood: a national cohort study. Lancet Child Adolesc Health. 2019;3:408–17.

21 Markopoulou P, Papanikolaou E, Analytis A, et al. Preterm birth as a risk factor for metabolic syndrome and cardiovascular disease in adult life: a systematic review and meta-analysis. J Pediatr. 2019;210:69–80.

22 Parkinson JRC, Hyde MJ, Gale C, et al. Preterm birth and the metabolic syndrome in adult life: a systematic review and meta-analysis. Pediatrics. 2013;131:e1240–63.

23 Lewington S, Clarke R, Qizilbash N, et al. Age-specific relevance of usual blood pressure to vascular mortality: a meta-analysis of individual data for one million adults in 61 prospective studies. Lancet. 2002;360:1903–13.

24 Crump C, Sundquist J, Sundquist K. Preterm birth and risk of type 1 and type 2 diabetes: a national cohort study. Diabetologia. 2020;63:508–18.

25 Thomas EL, Parkinson JR, Hyde MJ, et al. Aberrant adiposity and ectopic lipid deposition characterise the adult phenotype of the preterm infant. Pediatr Res. 2011;70:507–12.

26 Parkinson JRC, Emsley R, Adkins JLT, et al. Clinical and molecular evidence of accelerated ageing following very preterm birth. Pediatr Res. 2020;87:1005–10.

27 Weber M, Grote V, Closa-Monasterolo R, et al. European Childhood Obesity Trial Study Group. Lower protein content in infant formula reduces BMI and obesity risk at school age: follow-up of a randomized trial. Am J Clin Nutr. 2014;99:1041–51.

28 Modi N. The implications of routine milk fortification for the short and long-term health of preterm babies. Semin Fetal Neonatal Med. 2021;29(3):101216.

29 Qiu X, Lu JH, He JR, et al. The born in Guangzhou cohort study (BIGCS). Eur J Epidemiol. 2017;32:337–46.

30 Norris T, Ramel SE, Catalano P, et al. New charts for the assessment of body composition, according to air-displacement plethysmography, at birth and across the first 6 months of life Am J Clin Nutr. 2019;109:1353–60.

Neena Modi
Imperial College of London
Section of Neonatal Medicine, Faculty of Medicine
Chelsea and Westminster Hospital Campus
369 Fulham Road
London SW10 9NH
UK
n.modi@imperial.ac.uk

Published online: May 10, 2022

Embleton ND, Haschke F, Bode L (eds): Strategies in Neonatal Care to Promote Optimized Growth and
Development: Focus on Low Birth Weight Infants. 96th Nestlé Nutrition Institute Workshop, May 2021.
Nestlé Nutr Inst Workshop Ser. Basel, Karger, 2022, vol 96, pp 54–56 (DOI: 10.1159/000519402)

Summary on Optimizing Feeding, Nutrition and Growth on the NICU and after Discharge

The last 20–30 years have seen dramatic improvements in the survival of low birth weight (LBW) infants, especially those born preterm. In many neonatal intensive care units (NICUs) in well-resourced settings, it is common for preterm infants born more than 16 weeks early to survive. Many of these infants only weigh around 500 g and must accrete nutrients and grow at a fast rate during their stay on the NICU: at no other time in human life do we need to quadruple our weight in just 4 months in order to stay healthy. Clinicians must also consider the extreme nutrient vulnerability of such premature infants: body composition data show that around 85–90% of body weight at 24 weeks' gestation is water; in effect, this means clinicians must care for infants with only around 50 g dry lean mass. Further challenges are created by diseases such as necrotizing enterocolitis (NEC) and sepsis that are closely related to nutritional practices.

In the first session, Berrington considered the issue of starting and increasing feeds, milk tolerance and the monitoring of gut health. Whilst there are considerable data that suggest links between early feeding strategies and key short-term morbidities such as NEC and sepsis, there are few longer-term data. The majority of trials are underpowered for serious adverse outcomes like NEC, but recent large RCTs suggest there are no major differences on outcomes dependent on the speed of increases in milk feeds. The use of buccal colostrum to promote healthy oral microbiota and interact with the pharyngeal lymph node and immune system is increasingly practiced, yet there are few data from large trials. However, many clinicians consider this such a useful strategy, and it is questionable whether there is widespread equipoise that would deprive infants of this if early colostrum is available. Bloomfield and Cormack emphasized that whilst much greater attention has been applied to nutritional management in early life, there are still few data on the growth rates that optimize longer-term outcomes. Whilst nutrition is a universal requirement for all LBW infants, it is in many ways a relatively simple and inexpensive intervention, yet there are many weaknesses in the existing trials. This could be improved through the use of Core Outcome and Minimal Reporting Sets for nutritional studies. Embleton and colleagues considered the intimate link between nutritional exposures and brain growth in preterm infants. A more holistic concept of nutrition, beyond simply macronutrients and micronutrients was proposed that includes consideration of the functional components in milk feeds, the role of gut microbiota and sociotechnical (gavage feeding) and behavioral aspects (continued provision of expressed breastmilk) of nutrition. A range of different mechanisms that link nutrition to brain development were also discussed. Most obviously, sufficient macronutrients and micronutrients must be provided, but sufficient energy must also be provided in order to accrete those nutrients. Many nutrients may function through gene interactions (e.g., vitamin D) and others may have epigenetic effects such as DNA methylation that impact on aspects of growth and development. Human breast milk components may also impact on gut microbiota, that in turn impact on neurological function via the gut-brain axes. Finally, nutritional strategies that reduce diseases such as NEC, i.e. human breastmilk, will also improve brain outcomes via prevention of the "cytokine storm."

Haiden considered the complex issue of catch-up growth in preterm infants, and the importance of recognizing that nutritional needs of preterm infants should be considered as a continuum, from birth into later infancy. Dramatic changes in brain growth and processes take place in the first few postnatal months after term-corrected age. There are few studies that adequately explore the optimal timing of the introduction of complementary foods, but there are abundant data that emphasize the feeding difficulties many of these infants experience in early life. To meet these challenges, a multidisciplinary approach is needed. In the final talk of the session, Modi emphasized that whilst many opinions and authorities suggest that growth should mimic the pattern of a term born infant, there are no controlled trial data to support such an approach. Existing data show that body composition in preterm infants is profoundly different from that in term infants in early life, and there are also data to show that these differences exist in adulthood. Multiple factors impact on body composition and the quality of growth in early life, and these differences may be due to genetic and intrauterine exposures and influences. Modi concludes: "Progress in this area requires … high-quality, longitudinal cohort studies designed to … elicit causal inferences, and …[studies] of sufficient size to identify … functional outcomes … across the life course, be generalizable across populations, and have power to detect important interactions."

Nicholas D. Embleton

Published online: May 10, 2022

Embleton ND, Haschke F, Bode L (eds): Strategies in Neonatal Care to Promote Optimized Growth and Development: Focus on Low Birth Weight Infants. 96th Nestlé Nutrition Institute Workshop, May 2021. Nestlé Nutr Inst Workshop Ser. Basel, Karger, 2022, vol 96, pp 57–71 (DOI: 10.1159/000519400)

Donor Milk Banking – Safety, Efficacy, New Methodologies

Christoph Fusch[a, b]   Corinna Gebauer[c, d]

[a]Department of Pediatrics, Nürnberg General Hospital, South Campus, Paracelsus Medical School Nürnberg, Nürnberg, Germany; [b]Division of Neonatology, Department of Pediatrics, McMaster University and Hamilton Health Sciences, Hamilton, ON, Canada; [c]Human Milk Bank, Leipzig, Germany; [d]Division of Neonatology, Department of Pediatrics, University of Leipzig, Leipzig, Germany

Abstract

Donor milk (DM) is of increasing interest as primary nutritional source for preterm infants. Safe access requires special infrastructure, trained staff, sophisticated algorithms, and standard operating procedures as well as quality control measures. DM has limitations like low protein content and unpredictable composition of the other macronutrients, despite fortification frequently not meeting recommendations – both of them compromising growth. The first paragraph is devoted to COVID-19 and how it impacts processes of DM banking. The following paragraphs review aspects of "pasteurization," "safety audits/donor screening," and "DM nutrient variability." In summary, (i) Holder pasteurization still is the most suitable procedure for milk banks, but high-pressure pasteurization or ultraviolet C irradiation conserve the unique properties of DM better and deserve more research to make it suitable for clinical routine. (ii) In regard to safety/screening, guidelines are valuable for safe DM bank operation, but they differ between legislations. There is a surprisingly high rate of non-disclosed donor smoking (0.3%, $p > 0.05$) and of adulteration of delivered DM (up to 2%, $p < 0.05$) not detected by standard donor screening procedures. Frequencies differ between remunerated and non-remunerated programs. (iii) Neonatal caregivers should be aware of unpredictable composition of DM. They should be trained on how these can be overcome to avoid negative impact on growth and long-term outcomes like (a) measuring and disclosing nutrient contents of delivered DM batches to customers, (b) implementing certain types of donor pooling to reduce the risk of macronutrient depleted DM, (c) additional supplementation using 0.3–0.5 g protein/100 mL seems to be reasonable, (d) adjusted fortification may help to improve growth, but is not efficient in all preterm infants, (e) target fortification seems to improve growth (and probably also neurodevelopmental index) compared to standard fortification, (f) more research and clinical studies are needed.   © 2022 S. Karger AG, Basel

Introduction

Donor milk (DM) is of increasing interest as nutritional source for preterm infants, and on special occasions also for term infants. This interest is best reflected by a PubMed database search. For "donor milk," 30 publications were listed in 2008 with an exponential increase to $n = 205$ in 2020 and an extrapolated $n = 240$ for 2021. One-quarter to one-third of these papers refer to "donor milk banking" as improving the process, technology, and quality is key to providing safe and efficient DM for this very vulnerable population. In this state-of-the-art review about safety, efficacy, and new methodologies of DM banking, we will discuss three topics, namely "pasteurization," "donor screening," and "nutrient variability of donor milk" in more detail.

Currently, we are facing a worldwide SARS-CoV-2 pandemic that has touched nearly all aspects of human life and societies, so we would like to take the opportunity to start by having a look into how COVID-19 has impacted the work of human milk banks.

SARS-CoV-2

Impact on Pregnancy and Human Milk
What do we know so far about the risk of virus transmission to the fetus/newborn? A number of studies gives us the picture that in utero vertical transmission remains unproven [1–4] and transmission of SARS-CoV-2 due to vaginal birth appears unlikely [1, 3, 5, 6]. With respect to postnatal exposition, experience with other respiratory viruses suggested that it is unlikely that SARS-CoV-2 is transmitted via breastmilk [7, 8]. And in fact, until the time being there is no evidence of viable, infective SARS-CoV-2 in human milk [7, 9, 10]. On the other hand, SARS-CoV-2-specific immunoglobulin has been found in breast milk of infected mothers which might have a protective effect for the newborn [7, 8, 11].

Already early in March 2020, low rates of serious illness in SARS-CoV-2 infants were suggested by the evidence [12–14]. Isolating infants from COVID mothers and prohibiting breastfeeding was not associated with less postpartum virus transmission than with permitted breastfeeding plus appropriate infection prevention and control measures [15]. WHO recommended that "…in infants, the risk of COVID-19 infection is low and the infection is typically mild or asymptomatic. However, the consequences of not breastfeeding or separation of mother and child can be significant…" [16]. As a consequence, WHO published detailed recommendations on 13 March 2020 on the care of mothers and infants when maternal COVID-19 disease is suspected or confirmed [17]. Recommendations were coded regarding (1) skin-to-skin contact, (2) early initiation of breastfeeding, (3) rooming-in, (4) direct breastfeeding, (5) provision of expressed breastmilk, (6) provision of DM, (7) wet nursing, (8) provision of breastmilk substitutes (BMS), (9) psychological support for separated mothers, and (10) psychological support for separated infants [16, 17]. In short, WHO recommended no change in practice in all of the above fields.

Impact of SARS-CoV-2 on Practical Human Milk Management

Real life, however, is quite different. A recent study compared national versus WHO recommendations in 33 countries across the globe including all World Bank economic country groups [18]. The authors found poor adherence to WHO COVID guidelines regarding mother-newborn care and breastfeeding or DM use. Especially, there was low adherence with respect to mother-infant proximity/rooming-in (only 33 and 36%), indicating some substantial COVID fear. There was poor recommendation of access to DM with suspected or confirmed maternal COVID (12 and 9%). Adherence to expressed breastmilk recommendation was significantly higher (73 and 70%). The degree of deviation from WHO recommendations was not correlated with infant mortality rates or World Bank classified economic power.

Besides not adhering to WHO recommendations, common pandemic control measures were identified as roadblocks for DM supply [19]. Deferral of donors for 28 days in case of COVID-19 history was common practice despite different evidence. A study by the "Virtual Communication Network" which was established to collect data and experiences from milk banks across 35 countries provided an illustrative narrative review in which seven pandemic-related vulnerabilities in service provision were identified [20], amongst them DM availability. On one hand, DM demand was reported to have increased, mostly because mother's own milk (MOM) was quarantined for babies from COVID+ mothers. Other sources reported decreased demand because there was lack of knowledge that SARS-CoV-2 is inactivated by pasteurization (apart from that other research found out that there is no transmission via human milk at all). With respect to supply, there were different reports about a DH shortage, for instance because outside-the-hospital donations were shut down to avoid over-crowding, because donor numbers decreased due to fear of leaving the house and trying to avoid hospital visits, because of difficult access to test centers and phlebotomy services for screening. Supply was also impacted because basic transport infrastructures closed (e.g., ferry network in British Columbia; some air freight services where milk banks serve large geographical area) but also again for milk quarantining (i.e., 14 days after pasteurization kept frozen and release only after reassurance by phone that donor mothers kept symptom-free for the previous 14–28 days). However, from other authors there were also reports that DM volume increased during COVID times – from 63 to 113 L/month [21]. This is supported by personal observations that the percentage of mothers increased who are successfully nursing MOM in-hospital. COVID social distancing measures and in hospital visit restrictions seem to provide less distraction and disruption for mother-newborn pairs mostly because no one other than the father is granted access in most nursing units (pers. obs.).

SARS-CoV-2 and DM Supply
There are no detailed reports on how much SARS-CoV-2 impacted human milk bank functionality. Unpublished data from the DM bank from Leipzig, which is the largest one in Germany, indicate a two-step decrease in donations (by 40%) parallel to the lockdown activities (pers. commun. by Dr. Corinna Gebauer, Director of Donor Milk Bank, Leipzig). It is of interest to note that the demand for DM did not change despite reports that pandemic control measures might also reduce extreme prematurity (see Fig. 1).

In conclusion, SARS-CoV-2 should not affect DMB activities with respect to donor availability because it does not seem to be transmitted via human milk. However, pandemic control measures impact access to DM programs and pose a significant threat to the sustainability of DM supply.

Pasteurization: New Technology – Safety – Efficacy

The Role of Pasteurization
Pasteurization is a highly active research area in DMB operation. It involves new technologies and touches safety aspects of DM banking: pasteurization is needed to neutralize diverse germs (bacteria, virus, mostly Cytomegalovirus), and low-temperature long-time pasteurization also known as "Holder" is the most frequently used method. But it also involves aspects of efficacy: due to the energy applied to human milk, pasteurization can affect the integrity of valuable micronutrients, bio-factors, immunoglobulins, and cellular components that

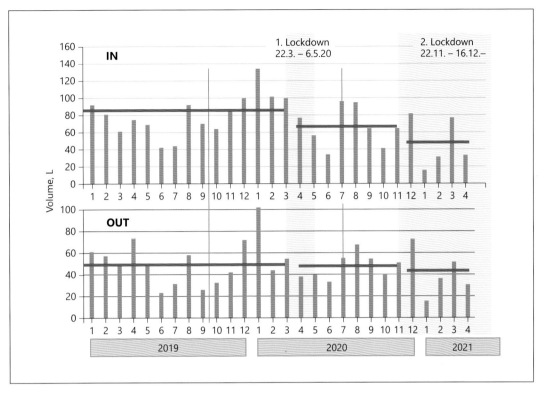

Fig. 1. Time course of donor milk supply and demand during the COVID-19 pandemic for the Human Milk Bank at the University Children's Hospital in Leipzig. Lockdown period during SARS-CoV-2 waves 2 and 3 are grouped together and marked as "2. Lockdown." It can be seen that lockdown activity decreased influx of donations, whereas the demand remained unchanged.

make human milk so unique [22–24]. It is common understanding that this cocktail should be preserved as much as possible. Though – on this occasion – it is of interest to note that for most of these factors, we currently do not exactly know what the biological meaning of these factors is. Do they play a specific role in preterm infants' gut health and growth or are they simply components of body fluids appearing in breast milk by transudation/passive transport/ultrafiltration? Regardless of this discussion, the process of pasteurization is an indispensable step for DM safety, and the challenge therefore is to find the appropriate equilibrium between amount and quality of energies applied.

SARS-CoV-2 and Pasteurization
To continue with the SARS-CoV-2 theme, it is of interest to note that standard low-temperature long-time Holder pasteurization inactivates SARS-CoV-2,

	LTLT	HTST	UV-C	HP-P
• Bedside/close to the unit	+ +	–	+ +	– –
• Training/skills required	+/–	+	+	+ +
• Microbial safety	+ +	+ +	+ +	+ +
• Virus elimination	+ +	+ +	+ (?)	???
• Nutritional value	– –	–	– –	–
• Availability	+ +	–	?	– – –
• Clinical evidence	+ +	?	?	?
• Costs	+ +	+ + +	+	+ + + +

Fig. 2. Summary of features of different pasteurization procedures. LTLT, low-temperature long-time pasteurization, i.e. "classical" Holder pasteurization; HTST, high-temperature short-time pasteurization; UV-C, ultraviolet C irradiation; HP-P, high-pressure pasteurization.

whereas cold storage down to –30 °C and 48 h does not [25, 26]. It is also of interest to note that these studies used artificially SARS-CoV-2 spiked BM samples because the virus is not naturally found in human milk.

Comparison of Pasteurization Procedures
While Holder pasteurization currently is the method of choice, there are other procedures under investigation. Of interest are (i) high-temperature short-time pasteurization (HTST-P), (ii) high-pressure pasteurization (HP-P) and (iii) ultraviolet-C irradiation (UV-C) pasteurization. While Holder uses 63 °C for 35 min, HTST-P applies T >72 °C for 15 s. HP-P uses pressures up to 500 MPsc (i.e., 5 × higher that the pressure present on the deepest point in the Pacific Ocean, the Mariana Trench) for several minutes at room temperature [27]. UV-C applies a wavelength between 200 and 280 nm for 10 to 50 s [28–30]. All methods eliminate bacteria and viruses, but conserve bio-factors to different degrees with HP-P and UV-C being the most promising ones (see Fig. 2) [31]. HTST-P and HP-P both need a special infrastructure, and the large-scale equipment requires a footprint that usually exceeds the capacity of most milk banks. Of interest to note that the research team of the milk bank in Warsaw (Poland) is developing a "miniaturized" HP-P device (U4000/86, Unipress, Warsaw, Poland) to reduce the burden on finances and space to make HP-P available for daily routine [32, 33]. A recent study confirmed that the combination of HP-P followed by freeze-drying may be a future way to process donated HM and make storage less complicated because technically freezers would not be needed any longer [32]. An alternative method worth exploring is the UV-C method because of its simplicity, efficacy, and conservation of bio-factors.

In conclusion, Holder pasteurization is still the most suitable procedure for most milk banks, but HP-P and UV-C conserve the unique properties of DM better and deserve more research to make it suitable in clinical routine for all milk banks.

Other Safety Aspects

Standard Operating Procedures
Safe operation of a milk bank is key. However, there are no uniform rules that regulate the day-to-day business. Differences are found between international regulatory authorities (like within the EU), between countries, but also between states/provinces/cantons of the same country. Working groups and professional associations have tried to establish manuals and textbooks describing common knowledge [34–40]. Study of this literature is highly recommended to all institutions in charge of either already running a milk bank or of planning to establish one. In this context, we would like to draw the attention to the recent study of Ben T. Hartmann from Australia who published a very thorough review about benefits and safety issues of milk banks [41]. Fourteen chapters list the potential hazards for all procedures and for all parties involved as donors, recipients, units, processes, and comment by providing the appropriate references. This review should be part of the inventory of contemporary milk banks.

Extended Donor Screening
Current practice is to screen first-time donor mothers for transmissible diseases in a similar way as it is done by blood banks and to repeat in regular intervals. This incorporates a thorough medical history as well as some laboratory and microbiological tests. Standard milk banks usually do not extend their screening beyond this point. However, there is a risk that donors smoke, take other medication, or consume (illegal) drugs without disclosing it to the program. Other undisclosed donor practices that jeopardize the quality of donated milk and may put recipients at risk are (i) dilution of DM with water, (ii) addition of non-human milk, or (iii) adding milk of a second donor. All these practices enhance the volume but deteriorate the quality and safety of DM and have been reported from programs that remunerate donors for the amount of delivered milk. But also in non-remunerated programs, it cannot be excluded that single donors follow such practice for a number of psychopathological reasons.

There is one paper that investigates the impact of extended donor screening, mainly by performing cotinine, medication, and drug tests, as well as tests to detect the presence of animal protein and of DNA other than from the registered donor's fingerprint [42]. The percentage of non-disclosed smoking was 0.3% and was not different between remunerated and non-remunerated programs (0.34 vs. 0.27%). There were no findings of illegal drug abuse or of other medication apart from 2 cases of oxycodone/oxymorphone in the non-remunerated program (9,439 samples tested) versus zero in the remunerated group (2,969 samples tested). The percentage of diluted samples, however, was significantly higher in remunerated donations (57 out of 2,875 samples tested, i.e. 2%) compared to 14 out of 2,060 samples tested in the non-remunerated program (0.7%).

In conclusion, a number of guidelines and reviews provide valuable information about safe operation of DM banks, but they differ between legislations. In DM programs, there is a surprisingly high rate of non-disclosed donor smoking (0.3%) and of adulteration of delivered breast milk (up to 2%) not detected by standard donor screening procedures. It needs to be decided whether a cotinine-positive rate of 3 out of 1,000 samples justifies the call for extended screening. Milk adulteration occurs more frequently but would be safely identified once macronutrient content of DM is measured and disclosed on a routine basis (see the section below).

Efficacy of DM: Suggestions for Improvement

Nutritional Physiology and Human Milk

Human milk is considered as the best nutritional source for preterm infants because (I) of the protein quality provided, (II) it contains bifido-promoting oligosaccharides, and (III) of a plethora of bio-factors and cellular components (whose role for preterm gut health is not fully understood yet). The disadvantage of human milk, however, is the low content of protein (P) and energy (E) which does not allow growth at rates that are appropriate for preterm infants of up to 21–24 g/kg/day. Such growth rates require intakes of 3.5–4.5 g protein and 120–160 kcal per kg and day – ideally in a balanced ratio of energy-to-protein (E:P). Comes on top that macronutrient levels vary within and between mothers and – what is even more important – the relationship between all macronutrients is highly variable as the mammary glands secrete carbohydrates, protein, and fat via different pathways. This means that there is no such thing as a more diluted or more concentrated human milk [43, 44]. In other words, human milk may provide all kinds of diets, balanced ones, but also diets with low-protein/high-fat or high-protein/low-fat or any other combinations that deviate from the optimum E:P ratio. Such unfavorable dietary intakes will jeopardize growth and potentially also neurodevelopment [45]. Unfortunately, no simple linear approach like increasing milk volume or standard fortifier strength above normal can cor-

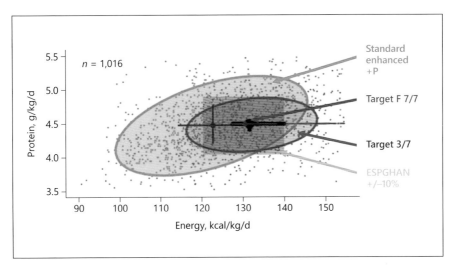

Fig. 3. Energy-to-protein plot for 1,016 breast milk samples from the double-blinded RCT on target fortification [46]. Three different fortification strategies are compared to improve deficiencies in nutrient intake after standard fortification. The colored dots represent all single values, the shaded areas represent the 95% limits for the distribution of each fortification strategy, the center dots with horizontal and vertical bars represent mean and standard deviations for both energy and protein. Green, standard fortification plus a fixed amount of extra protein (suggestion by I. Griffin in a letter to the editor [44]); blue, target fortification using milk analysis 3 times per week; pink, target fortification using milk analysis 7 times per week; maroon, ESPGHAN recommendations +/– 10%. It can be easily seen that linear fortification does not reduce the variability and leads to unpredictable dietary intake, whereas target fortification significantly reduces or eliminates this uncertainty. The degree of precision depends on the measurement frequency of milk composition. Reprinted from Rochow et al. [46] with permission from Elsevier.

rect "distorted" nutrient ratios and improve the efficacy of human milk. This is very nicely illustrated in a recent reply to letter to the Editor from our group (Fig. 3). As a consequence, concepts like target fortification (TFO) may be needed to overcome this significant problem [44, 46, 47].

DM and the Risk of Suboptimal Protein Supply
If preterm infants are fed DM, the risk of insufficient protein supply and postnatal growth faltering is even increased [48]. Protein content of DM is low because protein content drops during the first postnatal weeks to 0.8–1.4 g/100 mL, and DM is preferably obtained later in lactation [49]. Additionally, DM undergoes different handling steps like aliquoting, pasteurizing, freezing, thawing, and portioning to prepare daily feeds. The more frequently DM is handled the more macronutrients, especially fat (i.e., main determinant of energy), are lost to container walls [50]. There is an increasing number of publications that

confirm this fundamental deficiency of DM and report deficits in functional, mostly neurodevelopmental outcome [21, 51–55]. In fact, a recent study from Tufts University in preterm infants fed either MOM, DM or preterm formula (PTF) found that the DM group had the lowest Bailey scores at 2 years of corrected age [52]. This group also grew poorly compared to the groups receiving MOM or PTF.

Improved neurodevelopmental outcome was also not found in the most recent and most comprehensive RCT on the effect of DM in preterm infants known as the DOMINO trial [53]. A total of 299 preterm infants was randomized to receive either DM or PTF in case of insufficient mother's own milk supply. Demographics were not different between both groups. There was a statistically significant difference in NEC cases. However, there was no difference in the 18 months Bailey neurodevelopment scores. Also, there were no differences in growth rates between both groups. These results are somewhat unexpected and disappointing. It can be speculated that the beneficial effects of DM NEC protection on neurodevelopmental index (NDI) are being cancelled out by a negative effect of DM. The following paragraph shall try to interpret these findings and find a potential explanation.

The absolute difference of 4.8% NEC rate (6.8% in PTF vs. 2.0% in DM) should translate into improved NDI. It is reasonable to assume that the average NDI of a NEC patient is approximately 25 points below a normally grown non-NEC preemie, so the DM group should have improved by 175 points, i.e. + 1.2 per subject. However, table 2 of the DOMINO trial report shows that the DM group is approximately –2 NDI points below the PTF group (depending on the scores assessed, range of –1.6 to –3.0). Assuming that this delta of –3 NDI points is solely caused by nutritional differences (mainly protein) – and taking Stephen's relationship of protein intake and NDI into account – the DM group must have received –0.36 g/kg/day of protein less compared to the PTF group [54]. This figure corresponds favorably to the difference of protein concentration between donor and average native mother's own milk. According to the review by Embleton and van den Akker [55] about protein intake and growth rates, this delta of –0.36 g protein/kg/day would translate into a difference in growth rate of –1.8 g/kg/day. The DOMINO trial, however, was not powered to detect such differences. In conclusion, less nutrient supply and poorer growth in the DM group could still be an explanation for not finding an NDI difference despite a 70% drop in NEC rate.

Improvement of Macronutrient Content of DM
There are different ways to improve the quality of DM. First and foremost, it would be helpful that DM banks disclose the nutritional content of each single

batch they provide to neonatal units. Together with some education about nutritional physiology and growth NICU staff would be enabled to decide how ESPGHAN recommendations can be met with any given sample either by standard, adjusted, or target fortification, whatever would be the most appropriate and most simple approach to take. It is of interest to note that in a most recent paper by R. Lamb and coworkers from New Zealand it was stated that "…the variance in individual pooled DM indicates the importance of determining the nutrient composition of donated milk to inform fortification procedures…" [56]. Interestingly, DM banks in Poland measure macronutrient content using validated bedside methods and good clinical laboratory practice (GCLP) and disclose it to the unit (A. Wesolowska, pers. commun.) [57, 58].

Second, DM banks could start working on gradually reducing the variability of DM. This can be done by developing and evaluating pooling algorithms. A recent paper showed that multiple random pooling with up to 5 donors reduces the percentage of batches with critically low contents for both fat and protein. This can be improved by target pooling which requires prior knowledge of macronutrient content of all batches (i.e., best done by point-of-care analysis following GCLP [58]. These findings are confirmed by a study optimizing macronutrient content using different approaches and fortifiers [59].

A third approach would be to provide DM matched to gestational and postnatal age. The rationale is that protein content of human milk is high early in gestation and lactation – which to a certain extent parallels the requirements of preterm infants. There are some first clinical data on this concept available in a narrative review [21]. Protein content of DM can be as high as 2.1 g/100 mL which exceeds the average content of native human milk. With standard fortification adding some 1.1 g of protein per 100 mL, the ESPGHAN target of 3.0 g protein/100 mL could be reached. The study quotes better growth but does not provide detailed data. In summary, this approach looks promising. More clinical studies are needed. Needless to mention, this approach cannot fully compensate the risk of an unbalanced dietary E:P composition inherent in human milk either.

A fourth approach to improve macronutrient quantity and quality would be TFO. This concept acknowledges the fact of significant and unpredictable variability of macronutrient content of human milk. It attempts to correct imbalances by measuring macronutrient content of native breast milk batches, calculating potential deficits after standard fortification, and then adding appropriate modular nutrient components to reach ESPGHAN recommended intakes. TFO is not a super-fortification but identifies batches with insufficient nutrient content below standard assumptions and allows a more standardized macronutrient intake via breast milk. TFO is doable in clinical routine. The work to perform measurements of milk is similar to bedside or point-of-care analysis of blood gas samples – a procedure that no neonatologist would question. And subsequent preparation of milk batches is not fundamentally different from adding standard fortifier. It has been shown that TFO improves growth rates, and there is also a trend towards improved neurological outcome ($p = 0.07$); however, due to the relatively small sample size, the statistical significance is not reached at the 5%, but at the 7% error level (PAS/SPR annual conference 2018).

In conclusion, feeding human DM to preterm infants reduces NEC rates and feeding intolerance. In return, however, dietary supply with macronutrients is unpredictable on a daily level and may cause postnatal growth restriction and impact neurological development. Neonatal caregivers should be aware of these drawbacks inherent in breast milk physiology and be trained on how these can be overcome. Understanding this context may improve somatic and neurodevelopmental outcomes.

Summary – Improvement of Quality and Efficacy of DM
- Milk banks should measure the nutrient content of batches, improve pooling algorithms, and disclose the nutrient content of provided DM to the unit/customer.
- Certain types of donor pooling may help with avoiding macronutrient-depleted DM.
- In the meantime, additional supplementation using 0.3–0.5 g protein/100 mL seems to be reasonable [60].
- Adjusted fortification may help to improve growth, but is not efficient in all preterm infants. Data about NDI are not available.
- Data from our double-blind RCT show that TFO improves growth compared to standard fortification (most likely including NDI). It is precision medicine....
- This is confirmed by other recently published trials.
- More research and clinical studies are needed.

Conflict of Interest Statement

The authors declare no conflicts of interest. During the last three years, C.F. was invited as a speaker on conferences and/or had advisory roles with Medela, Nestlé, Hipp, Prolacta, Nutricia, Abbott, Hamilton. C.F. is a member of the executive committee of the Society of Neonatology and Pediatric Intensive Care (GNPI, Essen, Germany) and of the Human Donor Milk Bank Initiative (Frauenmilchbankinitiative, FMBI, Hamburg, Germany).

References

1 Marín Gabriel MA, Cuadrado I, Álvarez Fernández B, et al. Multicentre Spanish study found no incidences of viral transmission in infants born to mothers with COVID-19. Acta Paediatr. 2020 Nov;109(11):2302–2308.

2 Saadaoui M, Kumar M, Al Khodor S. COVID-19 infection during pregnancy: risk of vertical transmission, fetal, and neonatal outcomes. J Pers Med. 2021 May 28;11(6):483.

3 Juan J, Gil MM, Rong Z, et al. Effect of coronavirus disease 2019 (COVID-19) on maternal, perinatal and neonatal outcome: systematic review. Ultrasound Obstet Gynecol. 2020;56:15–27.

4 Walker KF, O'Donoghue K, Grace N, et al. Maternal transmission of SARS-COV-2 to the neonate, and possible routes for such transmission: a systematic review and critical analysis. BJOG. 2020 Oct;127(11):1324–1336.

5 Aslan MM, Uslu Yuvacı H, Köse O, et al. SARS-CoV-2 is not present in the vaginal fluid of pregnant women with COVID-19. J Matern Fetal Neonatal Med. 2020:1–3. doi: 10.1080/14767058.2020.1793318. Online ahead of print.

6 Wu Y, Liu C, Dong L, et al. Coronavirus disease 2019 among pregnant Chinese women: case series data on the safety of vaginal birth and breastfeeding. BJOG. 2020;127:1109–15.

7 World Health Organization Breastfeeding and COVID-19, 2020. Available from: https://www.who.int/publications/i/item/WHO-2019-nCoV-Sci_Brief-Breastfeeding-2020 [accessed 2020 June 23].

8 Chambers CD, Krogstad P, Bertrand K, et al. Evaluation of SARS-CoV-2 in breastmilk from 18 infected women. Preprint. medRxiv. 2020 Jun;2020.06.12.20127944.

9 Centeno-Tablante E, Medina-Rivera M, Finkelstein JL, et al. Transmission of SARS-CoV-2 through breast milk and breastfeeding: a living systematic review. Ann N Y Acad Sci. 2021 Jan;1484(1):32–54.

10 Lackey KA, Pace RM, Williams JE, et al. SARS-CoV-2 and human milk: what is the evidence? Matern Child Nutr. 2020 Oct;16(4):e13032.

11 Dong Y, Chi X, Hai H, et al. Antibodies in the breast milk of a maternal woman with COVID-19. Emerg Microbes Infect. 2020;9:1467–9.

12 Kam K-Q, Yung CF, Cui L, et al. A well infant with coronavirus disease 2019 with high viral load. Clin Infect Dis. 2020;71:847–9.

13 Wei M, Yuan J, Liu Y, et al. Novel coronavirus infection in hospitalized infants under 1 year of age in China. JAMA. 2020;323(13):1313–4.

14 World Health Organization. Report of the WHO-China joint mission on coronavirus disease 2019 (COVID-19), 2020. Available from: https://www.who.int/docs/default-source/coronaviruse/who-china-joint-mission-on-covid-19-final-report.pdf [accessed 2020 March 30].

15 Trippella G, Ciarcià M, Ferrari M, et al. COVID-19 in pregnant women and neonates: a systematic review of the literature with quality assessment of the studies. Pathogens. 2020 Jun;9(6):485.

16 World Health Organization. Clinical management of severe acute respiratory infection when COVID-19 is suspected, 2020. Available from: https://www.who.int/publications-detail/clinical-management-of-severe-acute-respiratory-infection-when-novel-coronavirus-(ncov)-infection-is-suspected [accessed 2020 May 27].

17 World Health Organization. Frequently asked questions: breastfeeding and COVID-19 for health care workers, 2020. Available from: https://www.who.int/docs/default-source/maternal-health/faqs-breastfeeding-and-covid-19.pdf?sfvrsn=d839e6c0_1 [accessed 2020 May 2].

18 Vu Hoang D, Cashin J, Gribble K, et al. Misalignment of global COVID-19 breastfeeding and newborn care guidelines with World Health Organization recommendations. BMJ Nutr Prev Health. 2020 Dec;3(2):339–50.

19 Jayagobi PA, Mei Chien C. Maintaining a viable donor milk supply during the SARS-CoV-2 (COVID-19) pandemic. J Hum Lact. 2020 Nov;36(4):622–3.

20 Shenker N, Staff M, Vickers A, et al. Maintaining human milk bank services throughout the COVID-19 pandemic: a global response. Matern Child Nutr. 2021 Jul;17(3):e13131.

21 Sánchez Luna M, Martin SC, Gómez-de-Orgaz CS. Human milk bank and personalized nutrition in the NICU: a narrative review. Eur J Pediatr. 2021 May;180(5):1327–33.

22 Picaud JC, Buffin R. Human milk-treatment and quality of banked human milk. Clin Perinatol. 2017 Mar;44(1):95–119.

23 Pitino MA, Unger S, Doyen A, et al. High hydrostatic pressure processing better preserves the nutrient and bioactive compound composition of human donor milk. J Nutr. 2019 Mar;149(3):497–504.

24 Peila C, Moro GE, Bertino E, et al. The effect of holder pasteurization on nutrients and biologically-active components in donor human milk: a review. Nutrients. 2016 Aug;8(8):477.

25 Unger S, Christie-Holmes N, Guvenc F, et al. Holder pasteurization of donated human milk is effective in inactivating SARS-CoV-2. CMAJ. 2020 Aug;192(31):E871–E874.

26 Walker GJ, Clifford V, Bansal N, et al. SARS-CoV-2 in human milk is inactivated by Holder pasteurisation but not cold storage. J Paediatr Child Health. 2020 Dec;56(12):1872–4.

27 Demazeau G, Plumecocq A, Lehours P, et al. A new high hydrostatic pressure process to assure the microbial safety of human milk while preserving the biological activity of its main components. Front Public Health. 2018 Nov;6:306.

28 Christen L, Lai CT, Hartmann B, et al. Ultraviolet-C irradiation: a novel pasteurization method for donor human milk. PLoS One. 2013 Jun 26;8(6):e68120.

29 Christen L, Lai CT, Hartmann B, et al. The effect of UV-C pasteurization on bacteriostatic properties and immunological proteins of donor human milk. PLoS One. 2013 Dec 23;8(12):e85867.

30 Lloyd ML, Hod N, Jayaraman J, et al. Inactivation of cytomegalovirus in breast milk using ultraviolet-c irradiation: opportunities for a new treatment option in breast milk banking. PLoS One. 2016 Aug 18;11(8):e0161116.

31 Peila C, Emmerik NE, Giribaldi M, et al. Human milk processing: a systematic review of innovative techniques to ensure the safety and quality of donor milk. J Pediatr Gastroenterol Nutr. 2017 Mar;64(3):353–61.

32 Jarzynka S, Strom K, Barbarska O, et al. Combination of high-pressure processing and freeze-drying as the most effective techniques in maintaining biological values and microbiological safety of donor milk. Int J Environ Res Public Health. 2021 Feb;18(4):2147.

33 Wesolowska A, Sinkiewicz-Darol E, Barbarska O, et al. New achievements in high-pressure processing to preserve human milk bioactivity. Front Pediatr. 2018 Nov;6:323.

34 Weaver G, Bertino E, Gebauer C, et al. Recommendations for the establishment and operation of human milk banks in Europe: a consensus statement from the European Milk Bank Association (EMBA). Front Pediatr. 2019 Mar 4;7:53.

35 Moro GE, Billeaud C, Rachel B, et al. Processing of donor human milk: update and recommendations from the European Milk Bank Association (EMBA). Front Pediatr. 2019 Feb;7:49.

36 Arbeitsgruppe Frauenmilchbanken Schweiz, Ahrens O. Leitlinie zur Organisation und Arbeitsweise einer Frauenmilchbank in der Schweiz. 2nd edition. Bern: Frauenmilchbanken Schweiz; 2020.

37 PATH. Strengthening human milk banking: A resource toolkit for establishing and integrating human milk banks. https://www.path.org/programs/maternal-newborn-child-healthandnutrition/strengthening-human-milk-banking-resource-toolkit/. 2019.

38 Centre for Clinical Practice at NICE (UK). Donor breast milk banks: The operation of donor milk bank services. NICE Clinical Guidelines, No. 93. London: National Institute for Health and Clinical Excellence (UK). https://www.nice.org.uk/guidance/cg93. 2010.

39 HMBANA Standards for Donor Human Milk Banking: An Overview. Public Version 1.0, September 2020. https://www.hmbana.org/file_download/inline/95a0362a-c9f4-4f15-b9ab-cf-8cf7b7b866 [accessed 2021 June 12].

40 Jones F. Best Practice for Expressing, Storing, and Handling Human Milk in Hospitals, Homes, & Child Care Settings. 4th edition. Fort Worth: Human Milk Banking Association of North America; 2019.

41 Hartmann BT. Ensuring safety in donor human milk banking in neonatal intensive care. Clin Perinatol. 2017 Mar;44(1):131–49.

42 Bloom BT. Safety of donor milk: a brief report. J Perinatol. 2016 May;36(5):392–3.

43 Fusch G, Mitra S, Rochow N, Fusch C. Target fortification of breast milk: levels of fat, protein or lactose are not related. Acta Paediatr. 2015 Jan;104(1):38–42.

44 Rochow N, Fusch C. Reply – Letter to the Editor – Individualized target fortification of breast milk with protein, carbohydrates, and fat for preterm infants. Clin Nutr. 2021 Apr;40(4):1463–6.

45 Henriksen C, Westerberg AC, Rønnestad A, et al. Growth and nutrient intake among very-low-birth-weight infants fed fortified human milk during hospitalisation. Br J Nutr. 2009 Oct;102(8):1179–86.

46 Rochow N, Fusch G, Ali A, et al. Individualized target fortification of breast milk with protein, carbohydrates, and fat for preterm infants: a double-blind randomized controlled trial. Clin Nutr. 2021 Jan;40(1):54–63.

47 Fabrizio V, Trzaski JM, Brownell EA, et al. Individualized versus standard diet fortification for growth and development in preterm infants receiving human milk. Cochrane Database Syst Rev. 2020 Nov;11(11):CD013465.

48 Quigley M, Embleton ND, McGuire W. Formula versus donor breast milk for feeding preterm or low birth weight infants. Cochrane Database Syst Rev. 2019 Jul;7(7):CD002971.

49 Gidrewicz DA, Fenton TR. A systematic review and meta-analysis of the nutrient content of preterm and term breast milk. BMC Pediatr. 2014 Aug;14:216.

50 Vieira AA, Soares FV, Pimenta HP, et al. Analysis of the influence of pasteurization, freezing/thawing, and offer processes on human milk's macronutrient concentrations. Early Hum Dev. 2011 Aug;87(8):577–80.

51 Perrin MT, Belfort MB, Hagadorn JI, et al. The Nutritional Composition and Energy Content of Donor Human Milk: A Systematic Review. Adv Nutr. 2020 Jul;11(4):960–70.

52 Madore LS, Bora S, Erdei C, et al. Effects of donor breastmilk feeding on growth and early neurodevelopmental outcomes in preterm infants: an observational study. Clin Ther. 2017 Jun;39(6):1210–20.

53 O'Connor DL, Gibbins S, Kiss A, et al. Effect of supplemental donor human milk compared with preterm formula on neurodevelopment of very low-birth-weight infants at 18 months: a randomized clinical trial. JAMA. 2016 Nov;316(18):1897–905.

54 Stephens BE, Walden RV, Gargus RA, et al. First-week protein and energy intakes are associated with 18-month developmental outcomes in extremely low birth weight infants. Pediatrics. 2009 May;123(5):1337–43.

55 Embleton ND, van den Akker CHP. Protein intakes to optimize outcomes for preterm infants. Semin Perinatol. 2019 Nov;43(7):151154.

56 Lamb RL, Haszard JJ, Little HMJ, et al. Macronutrient composition of donated human milk in a New Zealand population. J Hum Lact. 2021 Feb;37(1):114–21.

57 Fusch G, Kwan C, Huang RC, et al. Need of quality control programme when using near-infrared human milk analyzers. Acta Paediatr. 2016 Mar;105(3):324–5.

58 Kwan C, Fusch G, Rochow N, Fusch C; MAMAS Study collaborators. Milk analysis using milk analyzers in a standardized setting (MAMAS) study: a multicentre quality initiative. Clin Nutr. 2020 Jul;39(7):2121–8.

59 Fusch SF, Fusch G, Yousuf EI, et al. Fortification of breast milk: optimizing macronutrient content using different fortifiers and approaches. Front Pediatr, in revision.

60 Simmer K. Human Milk Fortification. Nestle Nutr Inst Workshop Ser. 2015;81:111–21.

Christoph Fusch
Children's Hospital, Nürnberg General Hospital
Department of Pediatrics
Breslauer Str. 201
DE-90471 Nürnberg (Germany)
Christoph.Fusch@klinikum-nuernberg.de

Published online: May 10, 2022

Embleton ND, Haschke F, Bode L (eds): Strategies in Neonatal Care to Promote Optimized Growth and Development: Focus on Low Birth Weight Infants. 96th Nestlé Nutrition Institute Workshop, May 2021. Nestlé Nutr Inst Workshop Ser. Basel, Karger, 2022, vol 96, pp 72–85 (DOI: 10.1159/000519397)

Meeting Protein and Energy Requirements of Preterm Infants Receiving Human Milk

Chris H.P. van den Akker[a]   Nicholas D. Embleton[b]
Marijn J. Vermeulen[c]   Johannes B. van Goudoever[a]

[a]Department of Pediatrics – Neonatology, Emma Children's Hospital, Amsterdam UMC, University of Amsterdam, Vrije Universiteit, Amsterdam, The Netherlands; [b]Newcastle Neonatal Service, Newcastle Hospitals NHS Trust, Newcastle upon Tyne, UK; [c]Department of Pediatrics – Neonatology, Erasmus MC – Sophia Children's Hospital, Rotterdam, The Netherlands

Abstract

Mother's own milk is universally recognized as the optimal source of nutrition for preterm infants, although most authorities agree a multi-nutrient fortifier must be added in order to support nutrient accretion at a rate comparable to in utero. Nevertheless, many preterm infants face a gap between achieved growth and what could have been achieved in utero. In this narrative review, we provide an overview on the macronutrient content in mother's own milk and donor milk and how this can be enhanced by the various available multi-nutrient fortifiers. We describe their general compositions and formulation, as well as several of their theoretical and practical advantages and drawbacks. In addition, differences between standardized fortification, or a more individualized approach like adjusted and targeted fortification are discussed. The optimal strategy however remains to be elucidated, and more experimental well-powered studies are therefore urgently needed. Until then, financial considerations and practical capabilities are likely to be the main drivers of local fortification strategies.

To facilitate nutrient accretion and growth in any individual, sufficient nutrition is of course required. Basically, this encompasses adequate amounts of protein of good quality, energy to finance the cost of protein synthesis, essential fatty acids, and all micronutrients including trace elements. Other requirements besides these nutrients are for example oxygen to facilitate energy generation, and anabolic hormones. The latter are, however, often suppressed in infants who are critically ill or inflamed, so that an anabolic state may be impossible to achieve.

Despite this basic knowledge, for many infants there is still a major gap between achieved growth in preterm infants admitted to a neonatal intensive care unit (NICU) and what would have been achieved on average if the fetus remained in utero. Although the incidence and severity of so-called extrauterine failure has decreased over the last decades, many infants at discharge have lost 1.2 standard deviations on average when compared to their birth standard deviation, as was shown in a recent report from 11 European countries [1]. In fact, 14% lost more than 2 standard deviations when compared to their birth z-score. On the other hand, there are also some reports typically from single centers that show this fall in the growth percentile can be prevented in the majority of preterm infants when paying meticulous attention to nutrition and growth [2].

In this narrative review, we will consider the various ways that the macronutrient intake in human milk-fed preterm infants can be improved. The discussion of adding specific bioactive factors (like for example human milk oligosaccharides, lactoferrin, vitamins, probiotics, enzymes, and hormones, etc.) is outside the scope of this review and can be found elsewhere [3]. All such factors may potentially interfere with nutrient availability, uptake, and utilization and therefore impact feeding tolerance and growth, either directly or indirectly. While there is a widely held belief that mother's own milk (MOM) from women delivering preterm contains more protein than from women that delivered at or close to term, there is actually only a clinically significant difference in the first few days after birth, as for example summarized in a systematic review on human milk nutrient content from a few years ago [4]. Furthermore, the protein content decreases rapidly after the first few weeks after which it stabilizes at around 1 gram per deciliter, both in human milk destined for either preterm or term infants. This finding was recently confirmed in the so-called "premature milk study," in which over 1,900 milk samples from 225 women were analyzed [5]. Whereas the interquartile range on milk protein content ranged from 1.0 to 1.5 g/dL at around postpartum day 10, these amounts decreased to 0.8–1.2 g/dL 4 weeks after birth. Outside the interquartile ranges, there is a much wider variation in nutrient content, which makes assumptions on nutritional intake in daily practice very difficult, if milk is not regularly measured for macronutrient content in a standardized way. Partly because of this wide variation, multi-nutrient fortifiers have tended to err on what might be considered by some to be the safe or lower side, in order not to provide too much protein or other nutrients. On average, typical powdered multi-nutrient fortifiers add about 1.0–1.2 g of protein to each 100 mL milk. If we convert what this protein content translates into daily milk consumption, one can infer that at around postnatal day 10, a preterm infant receives on average around 3.5–4.3 g protein per kg/day, an amount that would meet most recommendations which currently advise around 3.5–4.5 g/kg/day. However, after 4 weeks of age, when protein content in expressed milk is lower, the interquartile range of protein intake has decreased to about 3.2–3.8 g/kg/day after standard fortification. This might not be enough for many infants admitted at our NICUs if nutrient accretion similar to the intrauterine rate is the objective.

Protein Requirements

There are various different ways that protein requirements for preterm infants could be defined. First of all, one can take a factorial or theoretical approach. This simply involves determination of the amount of protein deposited in newly formed tissue at a growth rate that is similar to intrauterine. In addition, the amount of oxidized amino acids together with some inefficiency factors need to be added; also known as the obligatory nitrogen losses [6]. All-in-all, approximately 4 g/kg/day of enteral protein is assumed to be required to achieve a desired growth rate of 15–20 g/kg/day. However, as previously mentioned, this also depends on the availability of all other macro- and micronutrients as well as an optimal clinical condition.

Defining protein requirements can also be based on experimental evidence by providing more or less protein or multi-nutrient fortifier to human milk and assessing subsequent growth and other clinical outcomes. While the availability of the many very recent Cochrane reviews on human milk fortification for preterm infants may appear promising at deriving a scientifically based answer [7–12], the results are a little underwhelming. In the review by Brown et al. [7] on multi-nutrient fortification on human milk in general, for example, results on almost 1,500 preterm infants included in 18 trials are summarized. The authors concluded there were some modest increases in growth rates if human milk was fortified, and the lack of adverse effects of fortification were seen to be reassuring. On the other hand, no long-term benefits were demonstrated, although not unsurprisingly as it was only rarely reported and thus significantly underpowered. Besides that, there were several other limitations, in that for example the range of added protein was most often low (0.4–1.0 g/100 mL milk) and relatively old studies were included often with suboptimal methodological design. Besides, many studies also included moderately preterm infants (i.e., those above 32 weeks' gestation), were performed in low- and middle-income countries, or formula powder was used as fortifier rather than a specific human milk multi-nutrient fortifier.

Similar issues together with a lack of high-quality studies were encountered in the other cited Cochrane reviews, which make drawing firm and meaningful conclusions challenging. This means there are still several uncertainties around the use of multi-nutrient fortification of MOM or donor milk [13]. However, several cohort studies show that poor growth is associated with poor neurodevelopmental outcome [14, 15], and that these relationships remain valid after statistical adjustment from confounders like sepsis or necrotizing enterocolitis (NEC) or many other background variables. Other cohort studies, however, were less convincing at demonstrating such relationships [16]. Unfortunately, no large, high-quality, experimental randomized controlled trials (RCTs) in human milk-fed preterm infants have been performed. Thus, convincing evidence that more nutrients and better growth result in better long-term outcomes is lacking. However, there is some evidence from a highly cited RCT on preterm infants who were completely or partially formula fed to complement insufficient MOM [17]. In this trial conducted in the 1980s, over 400 preterm infants were randomized to receive in the first 4 postnatal weeks, either human milk supplemented with regular term formula if human milk was insufficient or unavailable, or a newly designed preterm formula with more nutrients in case of insufficient MOM. Following several years of follow-up, the study consistently showed that those in the intervention group not only grew better, but had persistently better neurological outcomes, up to the age of 16 years [18].

Multi-Nutrient Fortifiers

Since it is very clear that unfortified human milk results in poor postnatal growth, it is advised by for example the European Society for Paediatric Gastroenterology, Hepatology, and Nutrition (ESPGHAN) [19], the European Milk Bank Association (EMBA) [20], and the American Academy of Pediatrics (AAP) [21] that for all preterm infants a multi-nutrient fortifier is added to human milk. Various types of multi-nutrient fortifiers are theoretically available to choose from, as also depicted in Figure 1. The main composition of several available multi-nutrient fortifiers is outlined in Table 1. Comparisons of powdered with liquid fortifiers are slightly complicated due to the volume of human milk that is replaced by the fortifier. As such, in Table 2, nutrient content after mixing

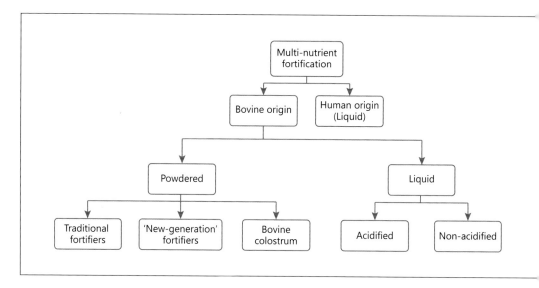

Fig. 1. Schematic overview of the various available types of multi-nutrient fortifiers.

the fortifier with preterm milk (with an average nutrient content) is calculated for easier comparisons. Practically, however, local availability of the different types or brands of fortifiers may be limited due to national legislation, registration, and allowance.

Multi-nutrient fortifiers typically contain currently at least 1 g of protein that is added per 100 mL of milk. The remainder is then made up of carbohydrates and sometimes lipids (vide infra) together with micronutrients, including electrolytes, vitamins, and several trace elements. The minerals phosphate and calcium, however, represent quantitatively the major contribution of the micronutrients and are essential in order to prevent metabolic bone deficiency of prematurity. In most of these fortifiers, the protein is of bovine milk origin. However, there is also a fortifier available that is produced from condensed donor human milk. Evaluation of the clinical advantage of a so-called human only diet requires large high-quality trials. Currently, only one RCT which studied this particular approach has been conducted so far [22], by comparing a standard multi-nutrient fortifier from bovine origin with a condensed human milk-based fortifier, and where both groups received donor milk in case of insufficient MOM availability. In this trial ($n = 125$), there were no differences in feeding intolerance as the primary outcome, nor were there differences in NEC stage ≥ 2, sepsis, or death, although there was less severe retinopathy of prematurity in the intervention group as a secondary outcome.

Table 1. Composition of selected multi-nutrient fortifiers

	Similac® HMF	Enfamil® HMF powder	PreNAN FM85® / Forti-Pré®/SMA® BMF/S-26® HMF	Aptamil® FMS/Nenatal® HMF/ Nutrilon® BMF/Almirón®/Fortema® / Cow & Gate nutriprem® HMF	Similac® HMF liquid	Similac® HMF liquid, hydrolyzed	Enfamil® HMF liquid	Prolact+ H²MF®
Manufacturer	Abbott	Mead Johnson	Nestlé / Wyeth	Nutricia/Danone/Milupa	Abbott	Abbott	Mead Johnson	Prolacta Bioscience
Formulation	Powdered	Powdered	Powdered	Powdered	Liquid; non-acidified	Liquid; non-acidified	Liquid; acidified	Liquid
Protein source, treatment, and type	Bovine; intact; whey	Bovine; hydrolyzed, whey	Bovine; partially hydrolyzed; whey	Bovine; extensively hydrolyzed; whey and casein	Bovine; intact; whey	Bovine; extensively hydrolyzed; casein	Bovine; partially hydrolyzed; whey	Human; intact; whey and casein
Typical ratio of fortifier with human milk (HM)	3.6 g; added to 100 mL HM	2.8 g; added to 100 mL HM	4.0 g; added to 100 mL HM	4.4 g; added to 100 mL HM	20 mL; added to 100 mL HM*	20 mL; added to 100 mL HM*	20 mL; added to 100 mL HM*	20–50 mL; add up with HM up to 100 mL**
Protein, g	1.0	1.1	1.4	1.1	1.4	2.0	2.2	1.2 (20 mL)
Carbohydrates, g	1.8	<0.4	1.3	2.7	3.2	3.0	<1.2	1.8 (20 mL)
Lipids, g	0.36	1.0	0.7	0	1.1	0.84	2.3	1.9 (20 mL)
Energy, kcal	16	14	17	15	28	28	30	29 (20 mL)
Calcium, mg	116	90	76	66	140	120	116	95 (20 mL)
Phosphorus, mg	64	50	44	38	80	68	63	53 (20 mL)

The list of available fortifiers may not be complete. Only the nutrients quantitatively most important are listed. Compositions are derived from manufacturer's leaflets. * Total volume after mixing is 120 mL. ** Total volume after mixing is 100 mL.

Table 2. Nutrient content per 100 mL of unfortified preterm MOM and multi-nutrient fortified preterm MOM, according to formulation and mixing instruction as outlined in Table 1

	Unfortified preterm milk*	Preterm milk fortified with:							
		Similac® HMF	Enfamil® HMF powder	PreNAN FM85®/ Forti-Pré®/SMA® BMF/S-26® HMF	Aptamil® FMS/Nenatal® HMF/Almirón® Fortema®/ Cow & Gate nutriprem® HMF	Similac® HMF liquid	Similac® HMF liquid, hydrolyzed	Enfamil® HMF liquid	Prolact+4 H²MF®
Fortifier to milk ratio		m/V 3.6/100	m/V 2.8/100	m/V 4.0/100	m/V 4.4/100	v/V 20/100	v/V 20/100	v/V 20/100	v/V 20/80
Protein, g/dL	1.2	2.2	2.3	2.6	2.3	2.2	2.7	2.8	2.2
Carbohydrates, g/dL	6.0	7.8	6.4	7.3	8.7	7.7	7.5	6.0	6.6
Lipids, g/dL	3.5	3.9	4.5	4.2	3.5	3.8	3.6	4.8	4.7
Energy, kcal/dL	67	83	81	84	82	79	79	81	83
Calcium, mg/dL	25	141	115	101	91	138	121	118	115
Phosphorus, mg/dL	13	77	63	57	51	78	68	63	63

* Average composition of preterm human milk expressed approximately 1 month postpartum [4, 5]. m, mass (g) of added powdered fortifier; v, volume (mL) of added liquid fortifier; V, volume (mL) of added unfortified human milk.

However, there are also significant challenges associated with the use of a condensed human milk-based fortifier. First of all, depending on the strength of applied fortification, 20–50% of MOM volume is displaced by current liquid human milk-based fortifier formulations. This leads to a significant reduction in the intake of beneficial bioactive factors present in fresh MOM, but which are much less abundant in the fortifier which is vat-pasteurized. Furthermore, the costs of this type of fortifier are high, and there are a range of organizational, societal, and logistical issues that might preclude widespread roll out of this type of product [23]. Therefore, large-scale trials independent of commercial funding and influence will be needed before this approach should be recommended. One such trial is the Swedish N-forte RCT (ClinicalTrials.gov: NCT03797157) where 222 preterm infants are included, and the primary outcome is expected to be complete early 2022. However, in order to prove a reduction in NEC, sample sizes in trials need to be much higher to gain sufficient power; for example, at least 862 infants are required to demonstrate a reduction in NEC rates from 10 to 5%.

Multi-nutrient fortifiers from bovine origin come in two forms; either powdered or as a liquid additive to MOM or donor milk. Due to the fear of contamination of powdered products with *Cronobacter sakazakii*, liquid fortifiers are available, and especially in the United States widely used. Liquid fortifiers have the advantage of complete sterility, either by heat treatment or acidification, which forms another distinction between these types (Fig. 1). Another benefit of liquid fortifiers is easier mixing. Yet, the main downside of liquid fortifiers is their volume replacement of MOM, typically a reduction of about 16.7% (% v/v = 20/120; Table 1). Furthermore, acidified liquid fortifiers have been associated with metabolic acidosis and poorer growth [24].

Powdered multi-nutrient fortifiers may be subdivided in the traditional or newer generation fortifiers. In more recent fortifiers, the amount of carbohydrates is reduced and replaced by lipids, which even form the largest caloric contribution (Fig. 2). These lipids are mainly in the form of medium-chain triglycerides, although essential fatty acids as well as the long-chain poly-unsaturated fatty acids (LC-PUFAs) docosahexaenoic acid, and arachidonic acid may be added in small amounts. This may help prevent a postnatal fall in LC-PUFA concentrations, although more research is needed to demonstrate if this is truly beneficial.

In order to increase the amount of bioactive factors in human milk, there is currently a trial being conducted, which adds powdered bovine colostrum to human milk as a new type of multi-nutrient fortifier (ClinicalTrials.gov: NCT03537365). Whether this approach can help reducing neonatal morbidities in preterm neonates, is to be awaited.

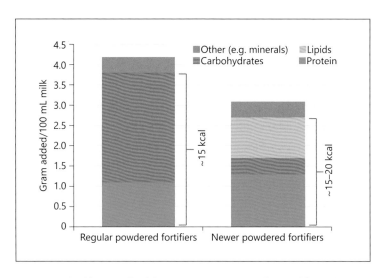

Fig. 2. Stacked bar graph of the main composition of typical formerly common and updated powdered multi-nutrient fortifiers which include lipids. Precise contents per brand are outlined in Table 1.

Fortification Strategies

As stated above, despite the various Cochrane reviews that have appeared in the last 2 years on human milk fortification [7–12], the evidence base on how to optimally fortify human milk remains relatively limited. On the other hand, there are also no consistent indications that adding fortifiers impairs gastrointestinal tolerance or other safety measures [25]. Once enteral feedings are tolerated after a few days of life, many clinicians choose to start to fortify MOM or donor milk, although the optimal timing (i.e., early or late introduction) in terms of growth or other clinical endpoints is understudied and thus unknown [8]. In addition, some clinicians and manufacturers prudently advocate to start with half-dose fortification as a precautionary measure, although scientifically, there is no reason to do so. Early and full-strength fortification not only increases macronutrient intake, but perhaps even more importantly, it may also aid to partially prevent or overcome early hypophosphatemia, which is frequently encountered in growth-restricted very preterm infants during the first week of life [26]. Similarly, on the other end, it is unknown when to stop multi-nutrient fortification: around discharge, several months after, or around a certain body weight. Simultaneously, practical issues become more important once the infant is partly or fully breast-fed, rather than fed with expressed milk.

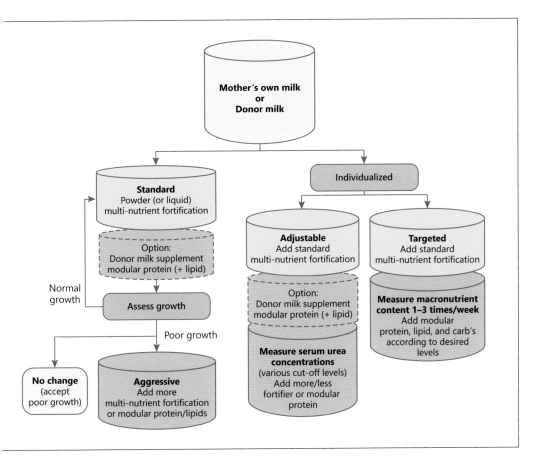

Fig. 3. Schematic overview of the various available strategies to fortify human milk for preterm infants. See main text for more details.

During multi-nutrient fortification, various approaches may be employed as is also graphically displayed in Figure 3. Classically, multi-nutrient fortification is protocolized in a standardized fashion according to manufacturer's instruction, although sometimes it may be topped up in case of suboptimal growth rates. Alternatively, fortification may be more individualized by adjusting according to measured serum urea concentrations or milk may be fortified to meet targeted macronutrient content goals after analyzing the milk. These approaches are also acknowledged by EMBA for example [20], but the optimal strategy remains to be elucidated [9]. Until then, financial considerations and practical capabilities are likely to be the main drivers of local fortification strategies.

Regardless of the employed fortification strategy as outlined in Figure 3, the first step always encompasses addition of a powdered or liquid multi-nutrient fortifier in amounts specified by the manufacturer (also depicted in Tables 1 and 2). In case donor milk is prescribed, some NICUs choose to add a standard extramodular protein supplement with or without extra modular lipids. This may replete the lower protein content of expressed human milk, amounting to around 1.0 g/dL or even less, when donated several months after birth to a milk bank [4, 27]. Similarly, due to the multiple container changes before milk arrives from the donor to the infant, fat content decreases slightly due to adherence to each of the several bottle walls. In addition, during classic Holder pasteurization of milk, for example bile-salt stimulated lipase and lipoprotein lipase are degraded almost entirely, which could hamper lipid digestion and uptake [27]. As such, standard modular lipid addition in the form of long-chain or medium-chain triglycerides may be warranted when relatively large volumes of donor milk are consumed.

In case of suboptimal growth despite standardized fortification, several options are available. One approach is to do nothing and accept poor growth, or one may increase total daily feeding volumes if tolerated gastrointestinally and by the current pulmonary and cardiac condition [28]. Modular protein with or without lipids may also be used as a top-on to promote growth as a more aggressive form of fortification. However, maintaining an appropriate protein to energy ratio is important to prevent oxidation of the majority of added proteins for energy production. We therefore recommended to monitor for high serum urea concentrations occasionally as a reflection of protein oxidation rather than anabolism, although safe and effective upper limits are unknown [29].

This latter approach partly resembles the so-called individualized adjustable fortification strategy, whereby default serum urea concentrations are measured, and fortification levels are either increased or decreased based on a relatively narrow bandwidth of serum urea concentrations. EMBA currently advises to maintain serum urea concentrations between 3.6 and 5.7 mmol/L (10–16 mg urea-N/dL, or 21–34 mg urea/dL) [20]. However, the evidence base for this tight range is very limited, and renal function or fluid status may make interpretations even more difficult. In addition, the recommended twice weekly urea measurements requiring blood are invasive and must also be considered.

Finally, a fully individualized approach when fortifying human milk, is the targeted approach [20]. This requires the analysis of the macronutrient composition of pooled expressed MOM or donor milk several times per week ideally, and the addition of modular protein, carbohydrates, and lipids on top of a standard multi-nutrient fortifier, to reach predefined levels. Obviously, this requires an appropriately calibrated milk analysis device and a dedicated nutritional team. On the other hand, by doing so, growth rates may be promoted, and there are some data to show they also result in increased fat-free mass, as shown in a recent RCT [30].

Conclusion

MOM is universally recognized as the optimal source of nutrition for preterm infants, although most authorities agree it must be fortified to support nutrient accretion rates comparable to in utero. Despite this, the optimal strategy of multi-nutrient fortification remains unclear due to a limited evidence base from high-quality controlled trials. More experimental well-powered studies are therefore urgently needed.

Epilogue

A potential downside of fortifying MOM that is often ignored by doctors is the psychological effect of all supplementation, as some mothers may feel that their milk may not be good enough for their child. This may hamper the motivation to continue expressing or giving breast milk after discharge, especially in mothers with additional mental health issues such as feelings of failure or guilt associated with premature birth [31]. It may also impact on health professional beliefs and attitudes towards breast milk: if we need to add so many nutrients, why not switch to formula feeding? It is therefore important to continually emphasize the advantageous components and effects of MOM itself, which are not lost during fortification and are of major benefit to the preterm infant.

Conflict of Interest Statement

C.H.P.v.d.A. reports participating in scientific advisory boards and giving lectures in educational symposia for Nutricia Early Life Nutrition, Baxter, and Nestlé Nutritional Institute.

N.D.E. reports research grants paid to his institution from Prolacta Bioscience and Danone Early Life Nutrition; and reports lecture honoraria from Nestlé Nutrition Institute.

M.J.V. is board member of the Dutch neonatal parent organization (Care4Neo) and of the National Breastfeeding Council; and participates in the scientific advisory board of Neobiomics; and reports grants paid to her institution from Nutricia – Danone.

J.B.v.G. is member of the National Health Council and founder and director of the National Human Donor Milk Bank in the Netherlands.

References

1 El Rafei R, Jarreau PH, Norman M, et al. Variation in very preterm extrauterine growth in a European multicountry cohort. Arch Dis Child Fetal Neonatal Ed. 2021;106(3):316–23.

2 Andrews ET, Ashton JJ, Pearson F, et al. Early postnatal growth failure in preterm infants is not inevitable. Arch Dis Child Fetal Neonatal Ed. 2019;104(3):F235–F41.

3 Mank E, Naninck EFG, Limpens J, et al. Enteral bioactive factor supplementation in preterm infants: a systematic review. Nutrients. 2020;12(10).

4 Gidrewicz DA, Fenton TR. A systematic review and meta-analysis of the nutrient content of preterm and term breast milk. BMC Pediatr. 2014;14:216.

5 Maly J, Burianova I, Vitkova V, et al. Preterm human milk macronutrient concentration is independent of gestational age at birth. Arch Dis Child Fetal Neonatal Ed. 2019;104(1):F50–F56.

6 van Goudoever JB, Vlaardingerbroek H, van den Akker CH, et al. Amino acids and proteins. World Rev Nutr Diet. 2014;110:49–63.

7 Brown JVE, Lin L, Embleton ND, et al. Multi-nutrient fortification of human milk for preterm infants. Cochrane Database Syst Rev. 2020(6):CD000343.

8 Thanigainathan S, Abiramalatha T. Early fortification of human milk versus late fortification to promote growth in preterm infants. Cochrane Database Syst Rev. 2020(7):CD013392.

9 Fabrizio V, Trzaski JM, Brownell EA, et al. Individualized versus standard diet fortification for growth and development in preterm infants receiving human milk. Cochrane Database Syst Rev. 2020(11):CD013465.

10 Premkumar MH, Pammi M, Suresh G. Human milk-derived fortifier versus bovine milk-derived fortifier for prevention of mortality and morbidity in preterm neonates. Cochrane Database Syst Rev. 2019(11):CD013145.

11 Amissah EA, Brown J, Harding JE. Protein supplementation of human milk for promoting growth in preterm infants. Cochrane Database Syst Rev. 2020(9):CD000433.

12 Gao C, Miller J, Collins CT, et al. Comparison of different protein concentrations of human milk fortifier for promoting growth and neurological development in preterm infants. Cochrane Database Syst Rev. 2020(11):CD007090.

13 Modi N. The implications of routine milk fortification for the short and long-term health of preterm babies. Semin Fetal Neonatal Med. 2021 Jun;26(3):101216.

14 Frondas-Chauty A, Simon L, Branger B, et al. Early growth and neurodevelopmental outcome in very preterm infants: impact of gender. Arch Dis Child Fetal Neonatal Ed. 2014;99(5):F366–F72.

15 Coviello C, Keunen K, Kersbergen KJ, et al. Effects of early nutrition and growth on brain volumes, white matter microstructure, and neurodevelopmental outcome in preterm newborns. Pediatr Res. 2018;83(1–1):102–10.

16 Fenton TR, Nasser R, Creighton D, et al. Weight, length, and head circumference at 36 weeks are not predictive of later cognitive impairment in very preterm infants. J Perinatol. 2021;41(3):606–14.

17 Lucas A, Morley R, Cole TJ, et al. Early diet in preterm babies and developmental status at 18 months. Lancet. 1990;335(8704):1477–81.

18 Isaacs EB, Gadian DG, Sabatini S, et al. The effect of early human diet on caudate volumes and IQ. Pediatr Res. 2008;63(3):308–14.

19 Moro GE, Arslanoglu S, Bertino E, et al. XII. Human milk in feeding premature infants: consensus statement. J Pediatr Gastroenterol Nutr. 2015;61(Suppl 1):S16–S9.

20 Arslanoglu S, Boquien CY, King C, et al. Fortification of human milk for preterm infants: update and recommendations of the European Milk Bank Association (EMBA) Working Group on human milk fortification. Front Pediatr. 2019;7:76.

21 Eidelman AI, Schanler RJ, American Academy of Pediatrics – Section on Breastfeeding. Breastfeeding and the use of human milk. Pediatrics. 2012;129(3):e827–e41.

22 O'Connor DL, Kiss A, Tomlinson C, et al. Nutrient enrichment of human milk with human and bovine milk-based fortifiers for infants born weighing <1250 g: a randomized clinical trial. Am J Clin Nutr. 2018;108(1):108–16.

23 Prouse C. Mining liquid gold: the lively, contested terrain of human milk valuations. Environ Plan A. 2021 Aug;53(5):958–976.

24 Schanler RJ, Groh-Wargo SL, Barrett-Reis B, et al. Improved outcomes in preterm infants fed a nonacidified liquid human milk fortifier: a prospective randomized clinical trial. J Pediatr. 2018;202:31–37 e2.

25 Ellis ZM, Tan HSG, Embleton ND, et al. Milk feed osmolality and adverse events in newborn infants and animals: a systematic review. Arch Dis Child Fetal Neonatal Ed. 2019;104(3):F333–F40.

26 Cormack BE, Jiang Y, Harding JE, et al. Neonatal refeeding syndrome and clinical outcome in extremely low-birth-weight babies: secondary cohort analysis from the ProVIDe Trial. JPEN J Parenter Enteral Nutr. 2021;45(1):65–78.

27 Colaizy TT. Effects of milk banking procedures on nutritional and bioactive components of donor human milk. Semin Perinatol. 2021;45(2):151382.

28 Travers CP, Wang T, Salas AA, et al. Higher- or usual-volume feedings in infants born very preterm: a randomized clinical trial. J Pediatr. 2020;224:66–71 e1.

29 Embleton ND, van den Akker CHP. Protein intakes to optimize outcomes for preterm infants. Semin Perinatol. 2019;43(7):151154.

30 Rochow N, Fusch G, Ali A, et al. Individualized target fortification of breast milk with protein, carbohydrates, and fat for preterm infants: a double-blind randomized controlled trial. Clin Nutr. 2021;40(1):54–63.

31 Palmquist AEL, Holdren SM, Fair CD. "It was all taken away": lactation, embodiment, and resistance among mothers caring for their very-low-birth-weight infants in the neonatal intensive care unit. Soc Sci Med. 2020;244:112648.

Chris H.P. van den Akker
Pediatrics-Neonatology
IC neonatology (H3)
Emma Children's Hospital - Amsterdam UMC
Meibergdreef 9
NL -1105 AZ Amsterdam
The Netherlands
c.h.vandenakker@amsterdamumc.nl

Published online: May 10, 2022

Embleton ND, Haschke F, Bode L (eds): Strategies in Neonatal Care to Promote Optimized Growth and Development: Focus on Low Birth Weight Infants. 96th Nestlé Nutrition Institute Workshop, May 2021. Nestlé Nutr Inst Workshop Ser. Basel, Karger, 2022, vol 96, pp 86–100 (DOI: 10.1159/000519394)

Human Milk Fortifiers for Preterm Infants: Do We Offer the Best Amino Acid Mix?

Ferdinand Haschke[a]   Johannes B. van Goudoever[b]
Nadja Haiden[c]   Dominik Grathwohl[d]

[a]Department of Pediatrics, PMU Salzburg, Salzburg, Austria; [b]Department of Pediatrics, Emma Children's Hospital, Amsterdam University Medical Centers, Amsterdam, The Netherlands; [c]Departments of Pediatrics and Clinical Pharmacology, Medical University Vienna, Vienna, Austria; [d]Nestlé Research Center, Lausanne, Switzerland

Abstract

For preterm and small-for-gestational age infants on enteral nutrition, the best solution is to add human milk fortifier (HMF) to human milk (HM) which is provided by the mother or a milk bank. HMF provides a means to add additional protein, energy, and micronutrients, while maintaining HM as the main source of nutrition. Because of their rapid increase of lean body mass, preterm infants have much higher protein requirements than term infants. Recommendations on protein requirements of preterm infants are available, but protein quality – i.e. the amino acid (AA) profile in HMFs has not been systematically assessed. Present guidelines for enteral nutrition recommend protein intakes around 4 g/kg body weight (BW) for preterm infants <1,500 g, an intake that is not achievable with unfortified HM intakes <200 mL/kg BW/day. It is generally assumed that the AA profile of HM is the best reference for the AA profile of HMF. We calculated advisable intakes of AAs for preterm infants between 400–2,500 g which are based on AA increments of the fetus. Corrections for absorption, inevitable losses, oxidation, and variation of AAs in HM were introduced. Our calculations indicate that extremely low birth weight (ELBW <1,000 g) and very low birth weight (VLBW <1,500 g) infants have substantially higher AA requirements than low birth weight (LBW) infants growing from 1,900 to 2,400 g. In ELBW infants, daily intakes of the different indispensable AAs (IAA) with 4 g of (term) HM protein/kg BW range between 59 and 125% of the respective advisable intakes. Intakes of 7 IAAs and 3 conditionally indispensable AAs (CIAA) are below advisable intakes. On the other hand, with 4 g HM protein per kg BW/day, the IAAs isoleucine and leucine and some dispensable AAs are already supplied in abundance. In VLBW infants, daily intakes of the IAA methionine and 3 CIAAs are still below the advisable intakes. In LBW infants (<2,000 g) receiving 3.5 g HM protein per kg BW daily intakes of 1 IAA and 3 CIAAs would be too low. Preterm infants should receive HMFs which provide adequate amounts of AAs which are needed for their rapid growth and development while avoiding excessive intakes. In particular, very high AA requirements of ELBW infants are a challenge. AA composition of present HMFs for preterm infants should be reconsidered: spiking HMF protein with the AAs which are presently undersupplied or providing targeted AA-based HMF are options to further improve the AA profile in fortifiers.

Protein and Amino Acids in Nutrition of Preterm Infants: What We Know and Need to Know

Mother's own milk is the first choice when enteral nutrition of extremely low birth weight (ELBW), very low birth weight (VLBW), and low birth weight (LBW) infants starts. Alternatively, banked human milk (HM) can be offered whenever mothers own milk is not available. HM has a strong trophic effect on the immature gut. This maturational effect not only enables earlier establishment of full feedings, it also provides protection against necrotizing enterocolitis (NEC) and late-onset sepsis [1] and has beneficial effects on brain development [2]. Proteins are an important constituent of HM, but also peptides and free amino acids (AAs) (5–10% of the total amount), molecules that also carry nitrogen atoms, are found in HM. All of these molecules can be used for tissue growth once absorbed. Besides their function as precursor for protein synthesis, HM contains many functional and immune-protective proteins and peptides [3–5]. Free AA are absorbed easily and may also serve a non-nutritive role as signaling molecules [6, 7]. Besides free AAs, peptides, and proteins, HM also contains non-protein-bound nitrogen such as urea molecules that may serve microbes in the intestines. In total, non-protein-bound nitrogen accounts for 20–25% of the total amount of nitrogen in HM.

Once full enteral nutrition is established or even earlier [1, 2], HM needs to be supplemented with HM fortifier (HMF) to meet requirements for growth. Because of their exceedingly high rate of growth, preterm infants, and specifically ELBW and VLBW infants have very high needs for all nutrients, among which protein is the most important one [2, 8]. After having adapted to extrauterine life and being in stable condition, these infants can grow as fast as the

Table 1. Gain [10, 28] and advisable intake of amino acids (AA) with fortified HM between 23 and 32 GW [6]

AA	AA gain, mg/kg/d			% AA gain	AA advisable intakes, mg/kg/d			AA in HM, mg/150 mL	% AA in HM	AA intake, mg/kg/d	Differences/advisable int./actual int. (AA), mg/kg/d		
	0.5–0.9	0.9–1.4	1.4–1.9 kg		0.5–0.9	0.9–1.4	1.4–1.9 kg	21–58 d		150 mL HM + 2.1 g HMF protein	0.5–0.9	0.9–1.4	1.4–1.9 kg
	23–26	26–29	29–32 GW		23–26	26–29	29–32 GW				23–26	26–29	29–32 GW
Indispensable AA													
(IAA)	(IAA)			(% IAA)	(IAA)			(IAA)	(% IAA)	(IAA)	(IAA)	(IAA)	(IAA)
ILE	84	62	52	9	176	130	109	97	13	220	44	90	111
LEU	181	133	112	20	380	279	235	178	24	403	23	124	168
LYS	174	128	107	19	365	269	225	123	16	278	−87	9	53
MET	49	35	29	6	103	74	61	27	4	61	−42	−13	0
PHE	101	74	62	11	212	155	130	69	9	156	−56	1	26
THR	101	74	62	11	212	155	130	82	11	185	−27	30	55
TRP	38*	28*	23*	4	80*	59*	48*	32	4	72	−8	13	24
VAL	115	84	70	13	241	176	147	100	13	226	−15	50	79
HIS	64	46	39	7	134	97	82	44	6	100	−34	3	18
Total IAA	917	664	556	100	1,903	1,394	1,167	752	100	1,701	−175	307	534
Dispensable AA													
(DAA)	(DAA)			(% DAA)	(IAA)				(% DAA)	(IAA)			
TYR	70	52	44	4	103	76	65	79	8	179	76	103	114
CYS	39*	29*	24*	2	57*	43*	35*	35	4	79	22	36	44
GLY	288	210	176	18	423	309	259	43	4	97	−326	−212	−162
GLU	317	231	194	20	466	340	285	302	31	684	218	344	399
ARG	186	137	114	11	273	188	168	67	7	152	−121	−36	−16
ALA	176	129	107	11	259	190	157	72	7	163	−96	−27	6
ASP	220	161	135	14	323	237	198	161	16	365	42	128	157
SER	107	78	65	7	157	115	96	80	8	181	24	66	85
PRO	205	150	125	13	301	220	184	150	15	340	39	120	156
Total DAA	1,608	1,177	984	100	2,362	1,718	1,447	989	100	2,240	−122	522	637
Total AA	2,515	1,841	1,540		4,265	3,112	2,614	1,661		3,941	−279	829	1,171
Weight gain g/kg/d	21	18	15										
Protein gain g/kg/d	2.5	1.8	1.5										

Differences between intake with HM + HMF (4 g HM protein/kg BW/day) and advisable intake. * Tryptophan [42] and * cysteine [35] were calculated from studies with stable isotopes.

fetus [9]. Daily protein gain/kg BW (kg body weight) of the fetus between 23–26 and 26–29 gestational weeks is about 2.7 and 2.0 times higher, respectively (Table 1, bottom line) than the protein gain of term infants during the first month of life [10–12]. As a result, a continuing challenge in the neonatal intensive care units is the need to nourish these infants to achieve healthy growth, often as much as 2–3 kg of body mass over a 12–16-week period. Rapid growth of lean body mass – for example muscle, bone, brain, and organ mass – cannot happen without the necessary high intakes of protein of high quality, since these organs are built on a protein matrix. Most importantly, brain growth and later life cognitive function are directly related to protein intake during the neonatal period in preterm infants. Although other factors such as illness may play a role in the causation of growth failure, inadequate intake of protein of the best quality can result in growth failure of the extent and with the consequences observed: growth failure is strongly associated with poor neurodevelopment and cognitive outcome, which has been well documented [13–15].

The recommendations on the amounts of protein needed by ELBW and VLBW infants [1, 2, 8, 16] are based on the reference fetus [11] and clinical trials which have recently been reviewed and form the basis of evidence-based guidelines [17]. The presently available powdered and liquid HMFs [18] deliver of 1.4–1.8 g/100 mL of milk and protein intakes are, therefore, nowadays close to the recommended protein target. The protein sources utilized for HM fortification are intact or hydrolyzed cow's milk whey fractions and casein. All cow's milk-based fortifiers on the market try to copy the AA profile of HM by spiking the fortifiers with AA. In addition, fortifiers which are based on HM protein came to the market during the last decade. However, the optimal protein quality in HMFs is still uncertain because it has not been systematically investigated [17]. The concept that the AA profile of HM is optimal for the rapidly growing premature infant was first challenged in a symposium on preterm nutrition almost half a century ago [19], on the grounds that protein requirements should not be separated from AA requirements. At that time, nothing was known about AA requirements of the preterm infant. Two recent studies which measured the protein concentration in HM provided to the VLBW and LBW infants indicated that delivering 1.4–1.8 g of fortifier protein with 100 mL of milk might still not be sufficient. [20, 21]. The authors of those studies speculated that the AA profile of the HMF which is close to HM is not perfect.

When aiming to meet all indispensable AA (IAA), conditionally indispensable AA (CIAA) [22], and dispensable AA (DAA) needs of preterm infants, in particular of ELBW and VLBW infants, the quality of the protein which is provided by HMF is important. It is assumed that the AA pattern in HMFs should be close to the pattern of HM protein. However, Fenton et al. [17] recently published evidence-based nutrition practice guidelines for preterm infants and concluded that no recommendations can be made on the quality of protein in HMF, because there are no studies in the literature. The quality of the protein may modify the recommended intake because the infant does not require protein but requires specific AAs. Individual AAs do not only serve as building blocks for protein synthesis and net protein balance [23], they also provide the basis for growth of all cells, tissues, and structural links between cells (e.g., dendrites among neurons), function as signaling molecules and neurotransmitters, and stimulate the secretion of growth-promoting hormones (i.e., insulin, insulin-like growth factor 1, IGF-1). If one or more of the IAAs or CIAAs become limiting for lean body mass gain and metabolism, specific body proteins may be degraded to free the limiting AAs. Consequently, the remaining AAs from the degraded protein become available as well and contribute to the excess of these AAs. They will be oxidized [24, 25] and thus serve as energy source (1 g = 4 kcal). AAs that are oxidized will yield ammonia, the source of urea, as well as CO_2. Especially during fetal life, AAs function as fuel source besides functioning as building blocks for protein. Following term birth, lipids become a more important source of energy. The increasing urinary urea nitrogen excretion in preterm infants during increasing protein supply may be due to their immaturity but may also indicate an increasing AA oxidation rate [26], suggesting a disbalance in the ratio of the supplied AAs [27].

Here, we reviewed the methods which were employed to measure protein and AA requirements of ELBW and VLBW infants. Moreover, we analyzed the available data on AA gains (increments) [10, 28] of the fetus between 23 and 40 weeks and present a mathematical model to calculate advisable AA intakes – in particular for ELBW and VLBW infants.

Amino Acids – Functions and Requirements

The specific roles, requirements, and metabolism of individual AAs and risks of deficiency have been described in detail [29]. As far as growth is concerned, all IAAs are fundamental for production of protein and key regulatory products. Especially leucine stimulates protein synthesis but, when provided in excess may become an important oxidative substrate [30, 31]. The branched-chain IAAs leucine, isoleucine, and valine, and the CIAA arginine stimulate insulin secretion, which in turn augments protein synthesis and protein accretion [32], but a recent Cochrane review [33] indicated that no clinical studies so far have been performed on the effect of branched-chained AA supplementation on growth of preterm infants. Lysine is primarily used for protein synthesis and a deficiency

Haschke/van Goudoever/Haiden/Grathwohl

in lysine intake, like for all essential AAs, limits protein synthesis and causes weight loss in young infants [34]. CIAAs and other DAAs are built from precursors (e.g., cysteine from methionine) but at present it is not clear under which conditions the formation of some CIAAs is limited in the preterm infant [29, 35]. Arginine, glycine, and proline require attention. Arginine is essential for ammonia detoxification through the urea cycle and is a precursor of nitric oxide, which is important for endothelial cell vasodilation and therefore for blood flow to growing organs. Preterm infants receiving low arginine intakes demonstrate elevated plasma ammonia levels and impaired nitric oxide synthesis during hypoargininemia [36]. Low arginine supply has been found to be associated with increased incidence of necrotizing enterocolitis [37]. A Cochrane review did indeed suggest that arginine supplementation may decrease the risk of necrotizing enterocolitis and the risk of mortality due to this disease [38]. Glycine, besides being a precursor of the major intracellular antioxidant glutathione, serves as an inhibitory neurotransmitter too. Enterally fed preterm infants, in particular SGA infants may have increased glycine requirements in case of oxidative injury such as during critical illness [22]. Proline is among the most abundant AAs in (connective) tissue protein (Table 1). Since preterm infants are unable to synthesize proline from glutamate and because of their high protein turnover and tissue accretion, they may have a particularly high proline requirement [22]. Glutamate, serine, and other DAAs promote fetal metabolism [22] and might be important for growth as well. Taurine is the most abundant free AA in HM but is not among the protein-bound AAs [6, 7]. It might contribute to development of brain function (vision, hearing), intestinal fat absorption, bile acid secretion. It is endogenously synthesized from cysteine, but at low rates in preterm infants. Despite the lack of evidence of a benefit from randomized clinical trials, taurine is considered to be a CIAA in preterm infants and is added to formulas for preterm infants and HMF.

AA requirements and metabolism of preterm and term infants can be studied by metabolic balance studies [38] and stable isotope techniques [23]. Balance studies are valuable and relatively easy to perform in larger groups of infants but are prone to errors because of their long duration when intake should be measured exactly, or additional errors as urine is sometimes difficult to collect and nitrogen may be lost through feces and skin. Furthermore, they do not specify intermediate metabolism or synthesis rates of certain AAs [22, 39]. The latter require stable isotope studies which can be performed safely in preterm infants [23]. The stable isotope technology has been employed to estimate protein turnover and requirements in rapidly growing premature infants who were appropriate or small for gestational age. Estimates of protein requirements were made based on measured turnover rates of the stable isotope-labelled AAs leucine and glycine [23]. Studies of AA requirements of LBW infants with those technologies are available in the case of phenylalanine, lysine, and cysteine [34, 35, 40, 41]. Phenylalanine requirements of LBW infants (>1.5 kg) were estimated to be 80 mg/kg/day (95% CI 40–119 mg/kg/day; [40]. Corresponding minimum requirements of term infants were 58 mg/kg/day (95% CI 38–78 mg/kg/day). Balance studies in VLBW infants [39] indicated a mean lysine retention of 291 mg/kg/day (weight 1.3, SD 0.2 kg), lysine requirements of term infants were 130 mg/kg/day [34, 41]. Thus, requirements in VLBW infants were approximately 2.2 times higher than those in term infants. If generous amounts of methionine are provided to LBW infants, <18 mg/kg/day of cysteine is required ($n = 25$; weight 1.78 kg, SD 0.32 [34]). It must be mentioned that estimates of phenylalanine, lysine, and cysteine requirements were established in LBW infants who were fed elemental formulas or preterm formulas under standardized conditions. Elemental formulas are known to yield higher AA oxidation rates than intact protein formulas. The weight of the LBW infants in those studies was between 1.3 and 1.8 kg. Therefore, information on AA requirements of ELBW/VLBW infants employing the stable isotope method and balance technology is scarce. Estimates on tryptophan requirements are available from 30 term neonates (gestational age 39±1 weeks) who were fed an elemental formula at 9±4 days. Mean requirement was determined to be 15 mg/kg/day (upper confidence interval 31 mg/kg/day [42]). In term infants during the first month of life, methionine (38 mg/kg/day; 95% CI 27–48 [43]), threonine (68 mg/kg/day; 95% CI 32–104; [44]), isoleucine (105 mg/kg/day), leucine (140 mg/kg/day), and valine requirements (110 mg/kg/day) have been published [45].

Calculating Advisable Amino Acid Intakes

We calculated advisable AA intakes (requirements) of ELBW and VLBW infants based on gains of the fetus. Such an approach has been established (factorial approach) for advisable protein- [11, 16] but not for AA intakes. Data on gain of fetal IAAs, CIAAs, and DAAs based on chemical analyses of 38 fetuses with gestational age between 11 and 40 weeks and birth weights 0.11–3.440 kg are in the literature [10, 28]. The data are good proxies to estimate how much of each IAA is required for gain of lean body mass and metabolism of the LBW infant. Data on tryptophan- and cysteine gains were not reported. We found that fetal protein content [10, 28] and therefore also protein gain between 28–40 weeks are very close to the reference fetus [11]. Employing curve fitting programs, we calculated best estimates for gains of IAAs (Fig. 1) and CIAAs/DAAs (Fig. 2) per kg BW. All AA gains declined in an exponential way with increasing BW. The con-

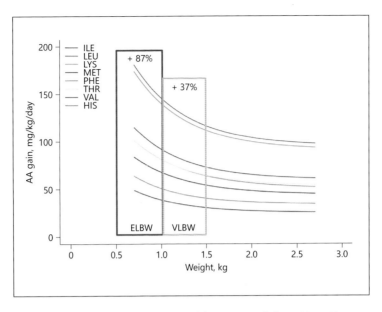

Fig. 1. Recalculated gain of indispensable amino acids from 23 to 40 gestational weeks [10, 28]. ELBW, extremely low birth weight infants; VLBW, very low birth weight infants.

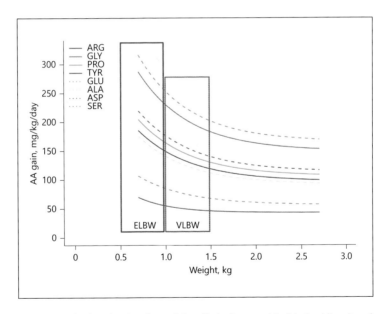

Fig. 2. Recalculated gain of conditionally indispensable (dashed lines) and dispensable amino acids (solid lines) from 23 to 40 gestational weeks [10, 28].

tribution of each AA to the increments in total AAs in the body did not change appreciably between 0.5 and 3.4 kg, which corresponds to the period of gesta tional age between 160 (approximately 23 weeks) and 280 days (term-equivalent age). This makes calculation of the advisable intakes of AAs based on gains much easier than they would otherwise be. Calculated daily gains of AAs/kg BW between 0.5–0.9 and 0.9–1.4 kg were approximately 87 and 37% higher, respectively, than gains between 2.4–2.9 kg. They were also 77 and 30% higher than of LBW infants growing from 1,900–2,400 g. Higher daily increments of AAs/kg BW of ELBW and VLBW infants are caused by higher weight gain/kg BW (Table 1, bottom line) but also by the fact that growth consists mainly of gain of fat-free mass [11]. After a BW of 1.5 kg is reached, weight gain rate becomes slower as the percentage of fat starts to increase in the body of the fetus. This is reflected in disproportionately lower increments of protein and AAs.

For calculation of advisable daily enteral intakes for each IAA/kg BW, we used the daily fetal gain as the basis requirement, added 30% to compensate for low absorption rates [39, 41, 46] and 20% for oxidation [46]. AAs which are delivered to the fetus are bypassing the intestine that is known to use AAs for (glycol)protein synthesis and as fuel. Consequently, fetal needs are lower than those of their corresponding enterally fed prematurely born counterparts [46]. For this reason, the advisable AA intakes were corrected for absorption and oxidation when calculated from AA gains in the fetus. 40% was added to compensate for inevitable losses [16, 18, 26, 39, 40]. Finally, we added 20% to compensate for assumed variation [7] of the AA concentrations in term HM. The calculated advisable intake of each AA corresponded to 210% of fetal gain. We assumed daily tryptophan requirements of ELBW infants to correspond to 2.5 times the upper confidence interval of term infants, which was established by the stable isotope method [42] and also corresponded to the intake with HM. For calculation of advisable daily enteral intakes for each CIAA and DAA (per kg BW), we first made an estimate how much could be synthesized in the body of preterm infants. The ratios of IAAs:DAAs (mg:mg) in the body between 0.5 and 3.4 kg BW are almost constant, around 2:1 (Table 1 [10, 28]). Corresponding ratios in milk of mothers who delivered preterm, as well as in transitory and mature HM of mothers who delivered at term are between 1.38–1.33 to 1.0 [6, 7]. Based on those calculations, we assumed that the preterm infants can synthesize at least 30% of DAA in the body and that 70% of AA gain is needed with enteral nutrition. The requirement for each DAA was therefore calculated as fetal gain (mg per kg BW/day) × 0.7. Corrections for absorption, inevitable losses, oxidation, and assumed variation of AA concentration in milk were made as described for IAAs. Cysteine requirement of ELBW was assumed to be 3 times the minimum requirement of LBW infants during the first month [35] and 60% higher than in term HM.

As the next step, we compared advisable intakes with those with HM without and with fortification. Table 1 shows published data on the amounts of AAs in 150 mL of "mature" HM, which corresponds to the amounts which an enterally fed premature infant usually receives/kg BW. We used the calculated data on AAs in "mature breast milk" of Zhang et al. [6] which are based on a systematic review of 26 articles providing 79 mean values from 3,774 subjects for total AAs in HM from a wide geographical distribution. Similar data on AAs in HM from several cohorts of Chinese cities were recently published [7]. Influences of gestational age and lactation stage were also reported in both studies. Calculated means for each AA in HM at different stages of lactation are available [6]. We selected the time interval 21–58 days after delivery ("mature HM"), because most donor milk provided is from that period of lactation or even later. Big differences between advisable intakes/kg BW and intakes with 150 mL of HM are evident both in the case of the IAAs and DAAs (Table 1). It can be seen that with HM, ELBW and VLBW infants do not receive the amount of each AA which would be needed for growth based on fetal gains. The data presented in Table 1 also indicate that the AA profile in HM does not match the profile of AA gains.

Reconsideration of Amino Acid Requirements during Fortification

To get an estimate of the daily IAA, CIAA, and DAA intakes of ELBW, VLBW, and LBW infants (per kg BW/day), we added those AAs (Table 1) which are provided by 2.1 g HM protein from HMF to the amounts in 150 mL term HM (21–58 days after delivery [6]) – i.e. total AA intakes are approximately 4 g/kg/day. Cow's milk-based HMF try to copy the AA profile of HM; therefore, AA intakes would be similar. In ELBW infants, daily IAA and total AA intakes with fortified HM are 175 and 279 mg/kg BW/day lower than the respective advisable intakes (Table 1). Corresponding cumulative intakes between a gestational age of 23 and 26 weeks (period of 21 days) are 3.7 and 5.9 g/kg BW lower. Intakes of 7 IAAs and 3 CIAAs are below the advisable intakes. IAA intakes range between 59 and 125% of the respective advisable intakes. As already mentioned, big gaps are caused by the high requirements of ELBW infants but also by differences between IAA profiles in HM and requirement profiles for fetal increments (Table 1). The biggest IAA and CIAA gaps between actual and advisable intakes are shown in Figure 3. In a preterm infant growing from 400–1,400 g the cumulative actual intake of lysine, which is important for protein synthesis [29, 34, 41] and the first limiting IAA in mammals, would be 1.6 g/kg BW lower than the advisable intake. HM protein provides only 16% of IAAs as lysine, whereas the contribution of lysine to the AA gains of the fetus is 19%. In VLBW infants, intakes

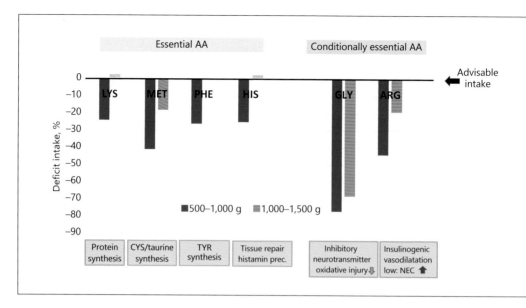

Fig. 3. Indispensable and conditionally indispensable amino acids: percent differences between advisable and actual intakes with 4 g human milk protein. Red columns indicate ELBW infants; yellow columns indicate VLBW infants. Functions of individual AA, see text.

of 1 IAA and 3 CIAAs are still below the advisable intakes, but leucine and isoleucine are already oversupplied. This indicates that the amounts and the profile of AAs in HMF for ELBW and VLBW infants need to be reconsidered. For the most vulnerable groups adequate intake of all AAs, in particular those which are indispensable, during the first period of life is key for normal growth and development as well as for long-term health. In LBW infants (i.e., infants >1,500 g), there are no more deficits in actual AA intakes if 4 g HM protein are provided (Table 1). However, if the recommended HM protein intake of 3.5 g for those infants [2, 8, 16] is provided, intakes of 1 IAA and 3 CIAAs are still too low. HMF which are based on cow's milk protein or HM protein should be spiked with those AAs where the intake might be too low. As an alternative, AA-based HMF could be developed which can provide tailor-made AA supply. We hope that quantity and profiles of AAs in HMF will be clinically studied in the near future. A tailor-made HMF should be offered in different concentrations to ELBW, VLBW, and LBW infants. However, development of HMF is costly because clinical trials are needed. Those trials are necessary to prove that the advisable intake based on AA gain of the fetus is safe and results in better growth and development than with the present HMF. On the other hand, business options are limited, because most neonatology departments are asking companies to receive HMF based on cow's milk protein fractions for free or at reduced costs.

Are Advisable Amino Acid Intakes for Preterm Infants Based on a Factorial Approach a Good Reference?

How solid is the estimate of advisable AA intakes based on AA gain in the fetus? (a) Fetal AA gains were published in the 70s of the last century. Chemical analyses of fetuses and stillborn infants would now only be allowed by ethical committees if the research is dedicated to disease prevention and treatment (e.g., cancer, HIV). Therefore, it is extremely unlikely that more data will be created and published. Widdowson's group accumulated a lot of experience in the field of chemical analyses of body components. Procedures and methods which were employed during tissue preparation and AA analysis [10, 28] correspond to today's practices. In addition, data presented to describe gains in fat and lean body mass and its components (e.g., protein, minerals) are close to the reference fetus [11] and therefore solid estimates. Her publication "The Chemical Composition of the Body" [47] is still a standard reference on AA in the human body. (b) It is likely that the AA pattern needed for growth and metabolism of ELBW/VLBW but also of LBW infants differs from that of infants born at term, because postnatal gains in weight and lean body mass/ kg BW are much faster. For those reasons, the needs of those protein fractions which are important for growth – mainly whey and casein – are higher, whereas it is not clear if the needs of non-nutritive proteins are higher as well [3–5]. Under such circumstances, the AA pattern in HM would not be the gold standard for preterm infants. (c) Strong support of the calculation of advisable intakes is provided in the case of lysine and phenylalanine by stable isotope research and metabolic balance studies [34, 40, 41]. The almost identical results that were derived from both approaches for those two IAAs, underline the strength of the reasoning. There is no reason to believe that the requirements should be far off for the remaining IAAs using our estimations. To be specific: our calculated advisable intake of lysine/kg BW is 2.1 times higher than the intake of term infants. Balance and stable-isotope studies indicated that lysine requirements/kg BW of VLBW infants are about 2.2 times higher than of term infants. Our calculation of advisable phenylalanine intake for LBW infants between 29–32 gestational weeks is 130 mg/kg/day. Stable isotope studies indicated that the upper confidence interval for minimal obligatory requirements of phenylalanine requirements for LBW (1.75, SD 0.17 kg; GA 32.5 weeks) was 119 mg/kg/day. Both lysine and phenylalanine are among the undersupplied AA by present HMF. Therefore, similar requirements found by 2 different methods support the request to increase concentrations of those IAAs in HMF, and (d) Banked HM is the backbone of enteral nutrition of preterm infants [48]. The AA profile of mature HM protein which was used in our calculations as an example for AA in HMF is realistic. Such HMF are on the market, and cow's milk-based HMF [49] try to have AA profiles which are close to HM protein.

Conclusions

Infants should receive HMFs which provide all amounts of AAs which are needed for their rapid growth and development. Our calculations which are based on AA gains of the fetus can serve as reference for advisable intakes of preterm infants. Very high AA requirements of ELBW infants are a challenge for enteral nutrition. AA profiles of present HMFs for preterm infants which are close to HM should be reconsidered: spiking HMF protein with the AAs which are presently undersupplied or providing targeted AA based HMF are options to further improve the AA profile in fortifiers.

Acknowledgements

The authors would like to thank Prof. E.E. Ziegler, University of Iowa, for reviewing the manuscript.

Conflict of Interest Statement

F.H. receives honoraria for lectures from the Nestlé Nutrition Institute and different nutrition companies. J.B.v.G. is founder and director of the Dutch National Human Milk bank and member of the National Health Council. Fees for consultancies and lectures are transferred to the Foundation that supports the Emma Children's Hospital. N.H. receives honoraria for lectures from Nestlé, Baxter, Danone, Novolac, and MUM. D.G. is an employee of Nestec Ltd, Switzerland.

References

1 Ziegler EE. Human milk – a valuable tool in the early days of life. Front Pediatr. 2019;2019:266.
2 Agostoni C, Buonocore G, Carnielli VP, et al. Enteral nutrient supply for infants: commentary from the European Society of Paediatric Gastroenterology, Hepatology and Nutrition Committee on Nutrition. J Pediatr Gastroenterol Nutr. 2010;50:85–91.
3 Haschke F, Haiden N, Thakkar SK. Nutritive and bioactive proteins in breastmilk. Ann Nutr Metab. 2016;69(Suppl 2):17–26.
4 Zhu J, Dingess KA. The functional power of the human milk proteome. Nutrients. 2019 Aug 8;11(8):1834.
5 Sánchez C, Franco L, Regal P, et al. Breast Milk: A source of functional compounds with potential application in nutrition and therapy. Nutrients. 2021 Mar;13(3):1026.
6 Zhang Z, Adelman AS, Rai D, et al. Amino acid profiles in term and preterm human milk through lactation: a systematic review. Nutrients. 2013 Nov;5(12):4800–21.

7 Garcia-Rodenas CL, Affolter M, Vinyes-Pares G, et al. Amino acid composition of breast milk from urban Chinese mothers. Nutrients. 2016;8:606–616.

8 Kleinman RE, Greer FR. Pediatric Nutrition. 7th ed. Elk Grove Village: American Academy of Pediatrics; 2014, pp 83–122.

9 Haschke F, Binder C, Huber-Dangl M, Haiden N. Early-life nutrition, growth trajectories, and long-term outcome. Nestle Nutr Inst Workshop Ser. 2019;90:107–20.

10 Widdowson EM, Southgate DAT, Hey EN. Body composition of the fetus and the infant. In: Visser HKA, editor: Nutrition and Metabolism of the Fetus and Infant. The Hague: Martinus Nijhoff; 1979. pp 169–177.

11 Ziegler EE, O'Donnell AM, Nelson SE, Fomon SJ. Body composition of the reference fetus. Growth. 1976;40:329–41.

12 Fomon SJ, Haschke F, Ziegler EE, Nelson SE. Body composition of reference children from birth to age 10 years. Am J Clin Nutr. 1982 May;35(5 Suppl):1169–75.

13 Ehrenkranz RA, Dusick AM, Vohr BR, et al. Growth in the neonatal intensive care unit influences neurodevelopmental and growth outcomes of extremely low birth weight infants. Pediatrics. 2006;117:1253–61.

14 Franz AR, Pohlandt F, Bode H, et al. Intra-uterine, early neonatal and post-discharge growth and neurodevelopmental outcome at 5.4 years in extremely preterm infants after intensive neonatal nutritional support. Pediatrics. 2009;123:e101109.

15 Biasini A, Monti F, Laguardia MC, et al. High protein intake in human/maternal milk fortification for ≤1,250 g infants: intrahospital growth and neurodevelopmental outcome at two years. Acta Biomed. 2018 Jan;88(4):470–6.

16 Ziegler EE. Meeting the nutritional needs of the low-birth-weight infant. Ann Nutr Metab. 2011;58(suppl 1):8–18.

17 Fenton TR, Griffin IJ, Groh-Wargo S, et al. Very low birthweight preterm infants: a 2020 evidence analysis center evidence-based nutrition practice guideline. J Acad Nutr Diet. 2021 Apr 2;S2212-2672(21)00149-0.

18 Ziegler EE. Equivalence of fortifiers. J Pediatr. 2019 Feb;205:291.

19 Visser HKA, Blom W, Van Gils JF, Zurcher T. Parenteral nutrition in low birth weight infants. In: Jonxis JHP, Visser HKA, Troelstra A, editors. Therapeutic Aspects of Nutrition. Fourth Nutricia Symposium. Leiden: HE Stenfert Kroese; 1973. vol 272.

20 Tonkin E, Miller J, Makrides M, et al. Dietary protein intake, breast feeding and growth in human milk fed preterm infants. Int J Environ Res Public Health. 2018 Jun 7;15(6).

21 Reid J, Makrides M, McPhee AJ, et al. The effect of increasing the protein content of human milk fortifier to 1.8 g/100 mL on growth in preterm infants: a randomised controlled trial. Nutrients. 2018 May 17;10(5):634.

22 Burattini I, Bellagamba MP, D'Ascenzo R, et al. Amino acid intake in preterm infants. Nestle Nutr Inst Workshop Ser. 2016;86:151–160.

23 Van Goudoever JB, Sulkers EJ, Halliday D, et al. Whole-body protein turnover in preterm appropriate for gestational age and small for gestational age infants: comparison of [15N]glycine and [1-(13)C]leucine administered simultaneously. Pediatr Res. 1995 Apr;37(4 Pt 1):381–8.

24 Hay WW, Thureen P. Protein for preterm infants: how much is needed? How much is enough? How much is too much? Pediatr Neonatol. 2010;51(4):198–207.

25 van den Akker CH, van Goudoever JB. Defining protein requirements of preterm infants by using metabolic studies in fetuses and preterm infants. Nestle Nutr Inst Workshop Ser. 2016;86:139–49.

26 Ridout E, Melara D, Rottinghaus S, Thureen PJ. Blood urea nitrogen concentration as a marker of amino acid intolerance in neonates with birthweight less than 1,250 grams. J Perinatol. 2005;25:130–3.

27 Kouwenhoven SMP, Antl N, Finken MJJ, et al. A modified low-protein infant formula supports adequate growth in healthy, term infants: a randomized, double-blind, equivalence trial. Am J Clin Nutr. 2020 May;111(5):962–74.

28 Widdowson EM. Chemical composition and nutritional needs of the fetus at different stages of gestation. In: Aebi H, Whitehead R, editors. Maternal Nutrition during Pregnancy and Lactation: A Nestlé Foundation Workshop, Lutry/Lausanne, April 26th and 27th 1979. Bern: Hans Huber; 1980. pp 39–48.

29 Kalhan SC, Bier DM. Protein and amino acid metabolism in the human newborn. Annu Rev Nutr. 2008;28:389–410.

30 Columbus DA, Fiorotto ML, Davis TA. Leucine is a major regulator of muscle protein synthesis in neonates. Amino Acids. 2015;47:259–70.

31 Van Veen LCP, Teng C, Hay WW Jr, et al. Leucine disposal and oxidation rates in the fetal lamb. Metabolism. 1987;36:48–53.

32 Gresores A, Anderson SM, Hood D, Hay WW Jr. Separate and joint effects of arginine and glucose on ovine fetal insulin secretion. Am J Physiol. 1997;272:E68–E73.

33 Amari I, Shahrook S, Namba F, et al. Branched-chain amino acid supplementation for improving growth and development in term and preterm neonates. Cochrane Database Systc Rev. 2020 Oct;10(10):CD012273.

34 Huang L, Hogewind-Schoonenboom JE, de Groof F, et al. Lysine requirement of the enterally fed term infant in the first month of life. Am J Clin Nutr. 2011 Dec;94(6)·1496–503.

35 Riedijk MA, van Beek RH, Voortman G, et al. Cysteine: a conditionally essential amino acid in low-birth-weight preterm infants? Am J Clin Nutr. 2007 Oct;86(4):1120–5.

36 van den Akker CH, van Goudoever JB. Defining protein requirements of preterm infants by using metabolic studies in fetuses and preterm infants. Nestle Nutr Inst Workshop Ser. 2016;86:139–49.

37 Amin HJ, Zamora SA, McMillan DD, et al. Arginine supplementation prevents necrotizing enterocolitis in the premature infant. J Pediatr. 2002;140:425–31.

38 Shah PS, Shah VS, Kelly LE. Arginine supplementation for prevention of necrotizing enterocolitis in preterm infants. Cochrane Database Syst Rev. 2017 Apr;4(4):CD004339.

39 Rigo J. Protein, amino acid and other nitrogen compounds. In: Tsang RC, Uauy R, Koletzko B, Zlotkin S, editors. Nutrition of the Preterm Infant: Scientific Basis and Practical Guidelines. Cincinnati, Digital Educational Publishing, 2005. pp 45–80.

40 Hogewind-Schoonenboom JE, Zhu L, Ackermans EC, et al. Phenylalanine requirements of enterally fed term and preterm neonates. Am J Clin Nutr. 2015 Jun;101(6):1155–62.

41 van der Schoor SR, Reeds PJ, Stellaard F, et al. Lysine kinetics in preterm infants: the importance of enteral feeding. Gut. 2004 Jan;53(1):38–43.

42 Huang L, Hogewind-Schoonenboom JE, Zhu L, et al. Tryptophan requirement of the enterally fed term infant in the first month of life. J Pediatr Gastroenterol Nutr. 2014;59:374–9.

43 Huang L, Hogewind-Schoonenboom JE, van Dongen MJ, et al. Methionine requirement of the enterally fed term infant in the first month of life in the presence of cysteine. Am J Clin Nutr. 2012 May;95(5):1048–54.

44 Hogewind-Schoonenboom JE, Huang L, de Groof F, et al. Threonine requirement of the enterally fed term infant in the first month of life. J Pediatr Gastroenterol Nutr. 2015 Sep;61(3):373–9.

45 De Groof F, Huang L, van Vliet I, et al. Branched-chain amino acid requirements for enterally fed term neonates in the first month of life. Am J Clin Nutr. 2014:99:62–70de.

46 van der Schoor SR, Wattimena DL, Huijmans J, et al. The gut takes nearly all: threonine kinetics in infants. Am J Clin Nutr. 2007 Oct;86(4):1132–8.

47 Widdowson EM, McCance RA, Spray CM. The chemical composition of the human body. Clin Sci. 1951 Feb;10(1):113–25.

48 Arslanoglu S, Boquien CY, King C, et al. Fortification of human milk for preterm infants: update and recommendations of the European Milk Bank Association (EMBA) Working Group on Human Milk Fortification. Front Pediatr. 2019 Mar 22;7:76.

49 Rigo J, Hascoët JM, Billeaud C, et al. Growth and nutritional biomarkers of preterm infants fed a new powdered human milk fortifier: a randomized trial. J Pediatr Gastroenterol Nutr. 2017 Oct;65(4):e83–e93.

Ferdinand Haschke
Department of Pediatrics PMU Salzburg
28 Müllner Hauptstrasse
AT -5020 Salzburg
Austria
fhaschk@googlemail.com

Published online: May 10, 2022

Embleton ND, Haschke F, Bode L (eds): Strategies in Neonatal Care to Promote Optimized Growth and Development: Focus on Low Birth Weight Infants. 96th Nestlé Nutrition Institute Workshop, May 2021. Nestlé Nutr Inst Workshop Ser. Basel, Karger, 2022, vol 96, pp 101–106 (DOI: 10.1159/000519398)

New Ways to Provide a Human Milk Fortifier during Breastfeeding

Nadja Haiden[a]   Ferdinand Haschke[b]

[a]Departments of Pediatrics and Clinical Pharmacology, Medical University Vienna, Vienna, Austria;
[b]Department of Pediatrics, PMU Salzburg, Salzburg, Austria

Abstract

Providing a human milk fortifier once the preterm infant has started to suckle at the breast can be challenging for the mother and might shorten duration of the breastfeeding period. Fortification is recommended up to term for the normal-growing infant and up to 3 months in growth-retarded infants. After hospital discharge, some mothers may not want to pump, fortify, and bottle-feed the fortifier-milk mixture any longer. They desire to breastfeed their infants directly from the breast, but unfortunately, fortification often interferes with direct breastfeeding. Cup feeding is the most researched fortification method and appears to be safe but cannot be applied during nursing. Another alternative is the supplemental nursing systems, but only a few low-quality studies investigated the method, which is difficult to handle and requires a lot of nursing experience. The use of a finger feeder to administer a fortifier to preterm infants is a new method that enables mothers to exclusively breastfeed their infants and meet their nutritional needs. Mothers reported easy preparation and handling of the fortifier. More than 67% of the infants accepted the device and fortifier application during nursing very well. However, the development of further methods to augment preterm infant nutrition that does not interfere with breastfeeding is of great interest. Future efforts to enable fortification during breastfeeding must be linked to the development of ready-to-use devices containing liquid human milk fortification mixtures.

The supplementation of human milk with human milk fortifiers (HMF) is a standard therapy for preterm babies during their stay in the neonatal units up until discharge. Breastfeeding is usually initiated as soon as possible but a coordinated sucking-swallowing-breathing pattern is not usually present before the infant's gestational age is 32 weeks [1] – at this time point, preterm infants start to take their first small-volume meals on the breast. Milk- and breastfeeding volumes increase with the strength and endurance of the infant which goes with neurological maturation that enables a more sufficient sucking-swallowing coordination. Breastfeeding should be encouraged at any time, but concurrent fortification while breastfeeding is challenging for mothers and their preterm infants especially during the early learning phase. Full breastfeeding is usually established around the term, which is also often the time point of discharge from the hospital. After discharge, the European Society for Pediatric Gastroenterology, Hepatology and Nutrition (ESPGHAN) recommends fortification of breast milk following the postnatal growth trajectory of the preterm infant. If weight gain after discharge continues to be above the 10th percentile, breast milk should be fortified until term gestational age. In the case of growth restriction, which is defined as weight gain below the 10th percentile, breast milk should be fortified up to 52 weeks' postconceptional age [2].

Cup Feeding

Cup feeding as a supplemental, alternative feeding method in the neonatal intensive care unit is a well-documented and safe method to apply HMF, but it affects direct breastfeeding [3]. A recent review investigated 12 studies on the safety and efficacy of cup feeding as an alternative, supplemental feeding method for breast-fed preterm infants [3] and found the method to be viable. When examining physiologic factors with cup feeding, it was illustrated through the 7 studies that cup feeding did not cause more physiologic distress than bottle feeding. The use of cup feeding resulted in a more stable heart rate and oxygen saturation than bottle feeding with similar weight gain. Additionally, breastfeeding rates were higher at discharge with continued higher rates at 3 and 6 months post-discharge for cup-fed infants [3]. Length of stay for cup feeding infants was found to be not significantly different between cup feeders and bottle feeders in 2 of the 3 studies that examined this variable. However, compliance to the intervention remains a challenge as cup feeding can not be applied during nursing [4] – the mother has to pump her milk, enrich it with a fortifier and feed it with a rather impractical cup device. Nevertheless, cup feeding may have some benefits for late preterm infants and improve breastfeeding rates up to 6 months of age [4].

Supplemental Nursing System and Supplemental Feeding Tube Devices

The supplemental nursing system (SNS) is a feeding tube device to provide babies with long-term supplemental feedings at the breast. When a baby is at the breast over a period of days or weeks, a hormonal mechanism is triggered that causes milk to be produced. It is used for inducing lactation, weak or ineffective "nursers," low milk supply, and premature babies [5].

Human milk fortification via an SNS has not been investigated yet, but fortifiers often attach to the walls of syringes and tubes, which might also be a problem here. Many mothers who used the device felt that it was difficult to use, and they needed assistance with it [6]. They also reported that the use of the device was time-consuming and cumbersome. Most women reported receiving help from the product instructional booklet beyond what they received from the lactation consultants and nurses. The other sources of assistance were from an experienced user or from the person who provided the device. Overall, the women had a strong desire to breastfeed and found the SNS an acceptable alternative method of supplementation, but these were mainly mothers of term infants [5].

Fortification Directly at the Breast by the Finger Feeder Method

Only a few studies investigated HMF application while breastfeeding in preterm infants after discharge. Each used a different method to administer the fortifier, one adding the entire dose into one bottle per day [7] with no adverse gastrointestinal symptoms reported, another was by the bottle but given spread out over the day [8], and the third by cup twice a day [9]. Again, these methods required pumping of breastmilk, which is uncomfortable for the mother and might hamper direct breastfeeding but none of the studies reported any adverse effect on breastfeeding rates in the fortified group. Fortifying breast milk for infants fed directly from the breast is logistically difficult and has also the potential to interfere with breastfeeding.

Recently, we investigated the acceptance, adherence, and feasibility of fortifier administration by finger feeder during breastfeeding [10]. Mothers were instructed (Fig. 1) and trained in fortifier application during breastfeeding by a lactation consultant before discharge and documented their experience via a self-reported feeding diary at home. Results of the observational study showed that the method was well accepted by 67% of the mothers. Mothers did not report problems in preparation or handling of syringes and finger feeder, but 33% of the infants stopped latching on or drooled milk during finger feeder use. Also, problems due to the bitter taste of the water-fortifier mixture were reported.

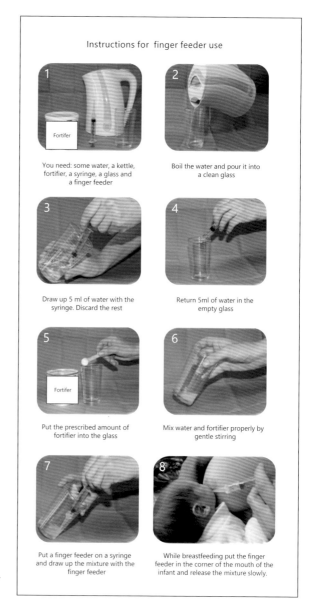

Instructions for finger feeder use

1 You need: some water, a kettle, fortifier, a syringe, a glass and a finger feeder

2 Boil the water and pour it into a clean glass

3 Draw up 5 ml of water with the syringe. Discard the rest

4 Return 5ml of water in the empty glass

5 Put the prescribed amount of fortifier into the glass

6 Mix water and fortifier properly by gentle stirring

7 Put a finger feeder on a syringe and draw up the mixture with the finger feeder

8 While breastfeeding put the finger feeder in the corner of the mouth of the infant and release the mixture slowly.

Fig. 1. Instructions for finger feeder use [10].

However, there was no effect on weight gain or growth of the infants in the group which used the fortifier (67%) in comparison to the group who stopped to use it due to problems (33%), which was surprising (Fig. 2). One can speculate that this observation is related to a lower milk intake induced by the higher caloric density of the fortified breastmilk, but this has to be investigated in further studies. Mothers who use feeder method positively remarked that they could stop pumping and feed directly from the breast. Medications such as multivitamin or

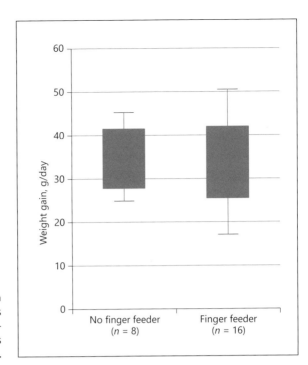

Fig. 2. Median weight gain in grams/day in infants whose mothers used the finger feeder and in infants whose mothers did not [10].

iron supplements, among others, could also be administered simultaneously with the finger feeder, which was also tolerated very well. The method appeared to be cost-effective because finger feeders and syringes are reusable products.

Fortification of breast milk directly during breastfeeding via the finger feeder method is an opportunity to cup or bottle feeding and does not interfere with breastfeeding. However, not all of the infants accepted the method. To avoid irritation for the infant, improvement in the flavor of the fortifier would be helpful. Multivitamin supplements, which are often prescribed, have a sweet taste. Splitting the daily dose of supplements into small portions might help sweeten the fortifier solution and make it tastier for the infant.

New Developments

Although the finger feeder method during breastfeeding is a further step towards exclusive breastfeeding in combination with fortifier application, there are still unsolved problems. The development of more user-friendly, ready-to-use devices or already prepared liquid fortifiers is of great interest. An already portioned and tastier product, which does not have to be pre-prepared is required. The need is to design a ready-to-use, disposable vial that contains one portion of liquid fortifier with an application tip so that the portion can be administered directly during breastfeeding.

In conclusion, the application of HMF during breastfeeding by finger feeder is a safe and feasible method, but further studies should evaluate effects on efficacy and growth. Future efforts should be linked to the development of ready-to-use, liquid HMF mixtures, which can be directly fed during breastfeeding.

Conflict of Interest Statement

N.H. receives honoraria for lectures from Nestlé, Baxter, Danone, Novalac, and MUM. No other conflicts of interest to declare.

F.H. receives honoraria for lectures from the Nestlé Nutrition Institute and different nutrition companies. No other conflicts of interest to declare.

Funding Sources

No funding was received for this work.

References

1 Newell SJ. Enteral feeding of the micropremie. Clin Perinatol. 2000 Mar;27(1):221–34, viii.

2 Aggett PJ, Agostoni C, Axelsson I, et al. Feeding preterm infants after hospital discharge: a commentary by the ESPGHAN Committee on Nutrition. J Pediatr Gastroenterol Nutr. 2006 May;42(5):596–603.

3 Penny F, Judge M, Brownell E, McGrath JM. Cup feeding as a supplemental, alternative feeding method for preterm breastfed infants: an integrative review. Matern Child Health J. 2018 Nov;22(11):1568–79.

4 Flint A, New K, Davies MW. Cup feeding versus other forms of supplemental enteral feeding for newborn infants unable to fully breastfeed. Cochrane Database Syst Rev. 2016 Aug(8):CD005092.

5 Penny F, Judge M, Brownell E, McGrath JM. What is the evidence for use of a supplemental feeding tube device as an alternative supplemental feeding method for breastfed infants? Adv Neonatal Care. 2018 Feb;18(1):31–7.

6 Chaturvedi P. Relactation. Indian Pediatr. 1994 Jul;31(7):858–60.

7 Zachariassen G, Faerk J, Grytter C, et al. Nutrient enrichment of mother's milk and growth of very preterm infants after hospital discharge. Pediatrics. 2011 Apr;127(4):e995–e1003.

8 da Cunha RD, Lamy Filho F, Rafael EV, et al. Breast milk supplementation and preterm infant development after hospital discharge: a randomized clinical trial. J Pediatr (Rio J). 2016 Mar-Apr;92(2):136–42.

9 O'Connor DL, Khan S, Weishuhn K, et al. Growth and nutrient intakes of human milk-fed preterm infants provided with extra energy and nutrients after hospital discharge. Pediatrics. 2008 Apr;121(4):766–76.

10 Thanhaeuser M, Kreissl A, Lindtner C, et al. Administration of fortifier by finger feeder during breastfeeding in preterm infants. J Obstet Gynecol Neonatal Nurs. 2017 Sep-Oct;46(5):748–754.

Nadja Haiden
Medical University of Vienna
Department of Clinical Pharmacology
Währinger Gürtel 18-20, AT -1090 Vienna (Austria)
nadja.haiden@meduniwien.ac.at

Published online: May 10, 2022

Embleton ND, Haschke F, Bode L (eds): Strategies in Neonatal Care to Promote Optimized Growth and Development: Focus on Low Birth Weight Infants. 96th Nestlé Nutrition Institute Workshop, May 2021. Nestlé Nutr Inst Workshop Ser. Basel, Karger, 2022, vol 96, pp 107–115 (DOI: 10.1159/000519392)

The Role of Long-Chain Polyunsaturated Fatty Acids in Very Preterm Nutrition

Andrew J. McPhee[a]   Carmel T. Collins[a, b]   Robert A. Gibson[a, c]   Maria Makrides[a, d]

[a]SAHMRI Women and Kids, South Australian Health and Medical Research Institute, Adelaide, SA, Australia; [b]Discipline of Paediatrics, Adelaide Medical School, Adelaide, SA, Australia; [c]School of Agriculture Food and Wine, The University of Adelaide, Adelaide, SA, Australia; [d]Adelaide Medical School, University of Adelaide, Adelaide, SA, Australia

Abstract

Infants born very preterm miss out on the in utero transfer of the omega-3 and omega-6 long-chain polyunsaturated fatty acids that occurs during the third trimester. A number of studies have explored the impact of increasing the enteral intakes of omega-3 +/– omega-6 long-chain polyunsaturated fatty acids to match fetal accretion rates in such infants. These studies have shown early transient improvements in vision and development with both strategies, but with the use of omega-3 supplementation alone appearing to increase the incidence of bronchopulmonary dysplasia. A recent study of omega-3 + omega-6 supplementation demonstrated a significant reduction in the incidence of severe retinopathy of prematurity in a high-risk population, without apparent adverse effects; a larger study is needed to confirm the observed benefits, to assess safety, and to determine long-term developmental outcomes of this strategy.   © 2022 S. Karger AG, Basel

Introduction

The omega-3 (*n*-3) long-chain polyunsaturated fatty acids (LCPUFAs) eicosapentaenoic acid and docosahexaenoic acid (DHA) together with the related omega-6 (*n*-6) LCPUFA arachidonic acid (AA) are felt to play important roles with respect to brain development and function (particularly vision), immune modulation, and the initiation and resolution of inflammation. Recognition of the fact that current feeding practices in very preterm (VPT) infants (<32 weeks' gestation), using either formula or breast milk, fail to meet the intrauterine accretion rates of LCPUFAs has prompted intense interest over the past 10–15 years as to whether LCPUFA supplementation aimed to match these accretion rates can improve neurodevelopmental outcomes and perhaps even favorably modify the diverse inflammatory morbidities of prematurity such as bronchopulmonary dysplasia (BPD), retinopathy of prematurity (ROP), necrotizing enterocolitis (NEC), and late-onset sepsis (LOS). This chapter reviews the results of randomized controlled trials that have addressed this issue.

Fats and Fatty Acids

Breast milk is the ideal food for infants. It has a high fat content which includes the essential *n*-3 and *n*-6 LCUPFA precursors, alpha linolenic acid (ALA, *n*-3), and linoleic acid (LA, *n*-6), respectively, as well as LCPUFAs such as DHA and AA. Breast milk DHA levels are largely determined by maternal diet, averaging 0.2–0.3% in mothers consuming a typical western diet, but increasing to >1% in populations with a high intake of fatty fish or DHA alone [1, 2]; on the other hand, breast milk AA levels are largely independent of maternal diet and average 0.4–0.5% of breast milk fats [1]. Although the essential fatty acids ALA and LA are present in breast milk and formula, and can be converted endogenously to their respective LCPUFAs, this process is thought to be limited in preterm infants, with the LCPUFAs thought to be conditionally essential.

The third trimester of pregnancy is a period of rapid growth, during which the fetal accretion rate of DHA via the placenta is estimated to be ~45 mg/kg/day and that of AA to be ~210 mg/kg/day [3]. Babies born very preterm miss out on the full benefit of this transplacental supply and have markedly lower levels of both DHA and AA in the week following birth [4], with the levels being directly related to gestational age, and with the levels decreasing further during the postnatal period [5, 6]. In this regard, lower levels of DHA following birth in VPT infants have been associated with BPD [5], while low levels of AA have been associated with LOS [5] and with ROP [6].

Recognition of the importance of the omega-3 fats, particularly in relation to retinal function, prompted studies of DHA supplementation in formula-fed term and preterm infants through the 1990s and early 2000s. These studies, which tended to involve more mature preterm infants and to exclude those with the typical problems of prematurity, supported beneficial effects with respect to visual function and neurodevelopment in both term and preterm formula-fed infants [7, 8]. Based on these studies, infant formulas were supplemented with DHA to match the average DHA content of western breast milk (~0.3% fats) beyond the early 2000s. Note that this level of supplementation results in a daily intake of DHA of ~15–20 mg/kg/day at a milk intake of 150–160 mL/kg/day); the comparable daily intake of AA based on a breast milk AA content of ~0.4–0.5% would be ~23–28 mg/kg/day. Obviously, these intake levels of both DHA and AA fall well short of their respective in utero accretion rates and likely explain the decrease in levels seen in VPT infants following birth and beyond.

Studies in VPT Infants Fed to Match in utero Accretion Rates of DHA +/– AA

Over the past 10–15 years, a number of randomized controlled trials in VPT infants have explored the impact of increasing the DHA +/– AA intake to approximate the in utero accretion rates seen in the third trimester. Outcomes of interest have included neurodevelopment and a number of the common morbidities seen in this population. These trials have included babies representative of the usual clinical profile for this group and have accommodated supplementation of both breast and formula-fed infants.

Henriksen et al. [9] randomized 141 infants born weighing <1,500 g to receive either mother's own or donor breast milk supplemented with 32 mg DHA and 31 mg AA per 100 mL compared to no supplementation. The intervention was started at 1 week after birth and continued until hospital discharge, with the primary outcome, cognitive development, being assessed at 6 months corrected age (CA) using the Ages and Stages Questionnaire. Subsequently, babies in the study had cognitive function tested at 20 months [10] and at 8 years of age [11]. In our DHA for Improvement of Neurodevelopmental Outcome (DINO) trial, we randomized 657 infants born <33 weeks' gestation to receive breast milk from their mothers who were supplemented with either 800 mg DHA per day (breast milk DHA ~1% of milk fats) or soy oil (breast milk DHA ~0.3% of milk fats); appropriate formula (1% DHA vs. 0.3% DHA, with no change in AA concentration) was available for use if mothers were unable to provide adequate amounts of breast milk [12]. The primary outcome, neurodevelopment, was assessed at 18 months [12] and at 7 years CA [13], with subgroups of children assessed for various functions at 4 months [14], 2 and 3–5 years [15], and at 7 years CA [16]. Moltu et al. [17] randomized 50 babies to milk supplemented to provide ~60 mg/kg/day DHA per day. However, this was part of a multicomponent supplementation strategy to increase energy, protein, vitamin A, and DHA intakes to reduce postnatal growth failure in infants weighing <1,500 g at birth; as such, it is difficult to tease out the effects, if any, of DHA alone in this study.

Our large N-3 Fatty Acids for Improvement in Respiratory Outcomes (N3RO) trial was specifically designed to determine the effect of DHA on BPD in infants born at <29 weeks' gestation [18]. The trial was designed to explore an observed secondary outcome of a reduction in the incidence of BPD (defined as an oxygen requirement at 36 weeks postmenstrual age; PMA) in boys (RR 0.67, 95% CI 0.47–0.96) and in infants with birth weight <1,250 g (RR 0.75, 95% CI 0.57–0.98) in the DINO study [19]. N3RO enrolled 1,273 infants and randomized them to receive either 60 mg/kg DHA per day via an enteral emulsion (n = 631) or a control (soy) emulsion without DHA (n = 642) from within 3 days of their first enteral feed and continuing up until 36 weeks' PMA or discharge home, whichever occurred first. The primary outcome was a diagnosis of physiological BPD at 36 weeks' PMA, as determined on the basis for supplemental oxygen or respiratory support with an assessment of oxygen saturation [20]. The parallel large Canadian study of Marc et al. [21], the Maternal Omega-3 Supplementation to Reduce Bronchopulmonary Dysplasia in Very Preterm Infants (MOBYDIck) trial, randomized breastfed babies <29 weeks' gestation to receive milk from their mothers who took supplements providing either 1,200 mg DHA per day or a 1:1 blend of soy and corn oils. The primary outcome was BPD-free survival at 36 weeks' PMA, with the diagnosis of BPD as determined in N3RO with the additional requirement for oxygen for at least 28 days. The MOBYDIck trial was terminated early, at 60% enrolment (high DHA n = 268; standard DHA n = 255), following publication of the N3RO results and an interim analysis of the MOBYDIck trial.

Two smaller Mexican studies of Bernabe-Garcia et al. [22, 23], explored the impact of DHA supplementation at 75 mg/kg/day compared to a sunflower oil control, given from day 1 of enteral feeding for 14 days, to babies with a birth weight of 1,000–1,499 g. In their first trial, 110 babies were randomized with a primary outcome of ROP incidence and severity [22], while in a later trial, 210 babies were randomized with a primary outcome of confirmed NEC [23]. Finally, the recent Mega Donna Mega study from the Swedish team of Hellstrom et al. [24] randomized 206 infants <28 weeks' gestation to receive either an enteral oil supplement containing 100 mg AA and 50 mg DHA/kg/day or no supplement from within 3 days of birth up until term, with the primary outcome being severe ROP defined as stage 3 and/or type 1 ROP.

Outcomes

Effect on Neurodevelopment and Visual Development
In the studies assessing neurodevelopmental and/or visual outcomes, some benefit of supplementation was seen in infancy, but not beyond 2 years. Thus, at 6 months of age (corrected for prematurity; CA), with 75% follow-up, the DHA/AA-supplemented infants of Henriksen et al. [9] showed better problem solving, while at 20 months, with a 65% follow-up, a significant improvement in attention was reported [10]; however, by 7–8 years of age, with 70% follow-up, no differences in cognitive outcomes were seen [11].

In the DINO study [12], although no difference overall was found in developmental quotient (DQ) scores at 18 months CA (follow-up 93%), less babies in the high DHA group had significant cognitive delay (DQ <70) (RR 0.50; 95% CI 0.26–0.93). In addition, girls randomized to the high DHA group had higher scores compared to controls (MD 4.5, 95% CI 0.5–8.5), and were less likely to have mild (DQ <85; RR 0.43, 95% CI 0.23–0.80) and significant cognitive delay (DQ <70; RR 0.17, 95% CI 0.04–0.72). In infants born <1,250 g, the incidence of mild cognitive delay was reduced in the high DHA group (RR 0.57, 95% CI 0.36–0.91). In exploratory post hoc analyses of the effect of maternal education and occupation, children in the high-dose DHA group whose mothers did not complete secondary education had significantly higher DQ scores (MD 5.3, SE 2.7; $p = 0.047$), as did those whose mothers were in trade, semi- or unskilled occupations (MD 5.6, SE 2.5; $p = 0.02$) [25].

In a subgroup of the DINO infants, there was no impact of high DHA on language development assessed at 26 months or behavior at 3–5 years CA [15]. Visual acuity in this group was better at 4 months CA [14], but in a different group of the DINO cohort, no long-term visual benefit was seen at 7 years [16]. By 7 years' CA, any early effect of high-dose DHA had washed out, though girls had poorer measures of executive function and behavior as reported by parents, but not as determined by objective psychological testing [13]. Inasmuch as there were only 200 babies <29 weeks' gestation in the DINO trial, the results of the neurodevelopmental follow-up of babies in the N3RO trial (at 5 years) and the MOBYDIck trial (at 2 years), will provide valuable information regarding the effect of high-dose DHA on cognitive function in those most at risk; these results are pending. Note however that in a small subgroup of the N3RO trial, assessment of attention at 18 months CA did not show any benefit attributable to high-dose DHA [26].

Effect on Mortality and Conditions of Prematurity
Mortality
There was no difference in mortality in any of the studies.

Growth
Although the Moltu study showed less growth failure in the group supplemented with DHA, the group was also supplemented with higher calories and protein, which likely explains the effect [27]. There was no effect of high-dose DHA (= /– AA) on growth up to 36 or 40 weeks' postmenstrual age in any of the studies that addressed this issue. With respect to growth beyond the neonatal period, babies in the high DHA group in the DINO study were significantly longer at 18 months corrected (82.8 cm SD 5.2; 81.7 SD 4.7, ratio of means 0.9 cm, 95% CI 0.2–1.2 cm), though with no effect on weight or head circumference [25]. In addition, those babies <1,250 g birth weight in the high DHA arm of the DINO study were longer at 4 months, heavier and longer at 12 and 18 months, and had a greater rate of head growth to 18 months CA compared to those with birth weight <1,250 g in the control group. Note however that the difference in head growth was small (0.017 cm/week, 95% CI 0.003–0.03 cm) [25]. By 7 years, there were no differences in any measure of growth or body composition between groups in the DINO study [13].

Bronchopulmonary Dysplasia
Although the DINO trial had suggested a reduction in BPD with an increased intake of DHA, the results of the N3RO study showed instead that high-dose DHA increased the incidence of physiological BPD in babies <29 weeks' gestation (RR 1.13, 95% CI 1.02–1.25, $p = 0.02$) [18]. Moreover, a similar finding was seen in the MOBYDIck study (RR 1.36; 95% CI 1.07–1.73, $p = 0.01$) [20], though no difference in the incidence of BPD was seen in the other, smaller studies, involving high-dose DHA (+/– AA). The mechanism via which high dose DHA may increase the risk of BPD is unclear, though studies in a neonatal murine model of BPD suggest that both the DHA metabolite, resolvin D1 and the AA metabolite, lipoxin A4 are beneficial in ameliorating lung injury [28]. Inasmuch as high-dose DHA supplementation results in a modest decrease in AA levels [18], it is possible that this limits the availability of AA metabolites, thus decreasing any benefit attributable to DHA. A pending analysis of LCPUFA metabolites from the N3RO study may help to clarify this issue.

Retinopathy of Prematurity
The Mega Donna Mega study was designed with severe ROP (defined as either stage 3 or zone 1 ROP) as its primary outcome [24] based on knowledge that the

DHA metabolite resolvin D1 inhibits neovascularization in a neonatal mouse model of ROP [29] and an association between low levels of AA in VPT and ROP [6]. The study showed a significant reduction in the incidence of this serious eye problem – RR 0.50; 95% CI 0.28–0.91, $p = 0.02$. High-dose DHA (+/– AA) had no impact on ROP in any of the other studies, apart from a lower rate of diagnosed grade 3 ROP with DHA supplementation reported in the study of Bernabe-Garcia et al. [22], though with no difference in the incidence of ROP overall and no difference in the need for intervention.

Other Conditions of Prematurity

There was no difference in the reported incidence of NEC in any of the studies apart from the 2021 study of Bernabe-Garcia et al. [23] in which high DHA supplementation for 2 weeks was associated with a reduction in the risk of confirmed NEC in babies with birth weight 1,000–1,499 g (RR 0.93; 95% CI 0.88–0.98). It is difficult to reconcile these results, in a relatively low risk population, to those from studies with much larger numbers of smaller and more immature babies. With respect to severe intraventricular hemorrhage (IVH) (defined as grade 3 or 4), high-dose DHA in the MOBYDIck trial was associated with a lower risk of severe IVH (RR 0.48; 95% CI 0.29–0.08) [21]; however, this is likely a chance observation, given that severe IVH typically has its onset in the first 3–5 days, yet the trial intervention was only just starting at this time in the study. There was no evidence of an impact of high DHA (+/– AA) on IVH in any of the other studies. Finally, there was an increase in the rate of LOS in the DHA-supplemented group in the study by Moltu et al. [17], though the authors attributed this to the higher dose of amino acids in this group. There was no difference in the incidence of LOS in any of the other studies in which it was recorded.

Implications for Clinical Practice and Future Research

Based on this review of studies aimed at providing DHA (+/– AA) intakes to VPT infants that approximate calculated in utero accretion rates, there appears to be consistent evidence of early developmental benefits, though with these not evident beyond 2–3 years of age and with the suggestion of an adverse impact of high DHA exposure on executive function in girls at 7 years of age. Long-term developmental follow-up, particularly of the large N3RO and MOBYDIck studies, may help to clarify this issue. High intakes of DHA alone appear to increase the risk of BPD, though do not appear to have any effect on mortality, ROP, IVH, LOS, or long-term growth. The impressive reduction in the incidence of severe ROP seen with the combined DHA + AA strategy in the Mega Donna Mega study requires confirmation with a larger study, which would also help to address safety issues, particularly with respect to BPD, and to assess long-term developmental outcomes.

Acknowledgements

Supported by Australian National Health and Medical Research Council Fellowships (Translating Research into Practice Fellowship [AAP1132596] to Dr. Collins, Senior Principal Research Fellowship [APP1046207] to Dr. Gibson, and Principal Research Fellowship [APP1154912] to Dr. Makrides).

Conflict of Interest Statement

All authors report grants from the Australian National Health and Medical Research Council (NHMRC). The views expressed herein are solely the responsibility of the authors and do not reflect the views of the NH and MRC. Dr. Gibson has a patent – "Stabilising and Analysing Fatty Acids in a Biological Sample Stored on Solid Media" licensed to Adelaide Research and Innovation, The University of Adelaide.

References

1 Brenna JT, Varamini B, Jensen RG, et al. Docosahexaenoic acid and arachidonic acid concentrations in human breast milk worldwide. Am J Clin Nutr. 2007;85:1457–64.

2 Makrides M, Neumann MA, Gibson RA. Effect of maternal docosahexaenoic acid (DHA) supplementation on breast milk composition. Eur J Clin Nutr. 1996;50:352–7.

3 Lapillonne A, Groh-Wargo S, Gonzalez CHL, Uauy R. Lipid needs of preterm infants: updated recommendations. J Pediatr. 2013;162:S37–S47.

4 Baack ML, Puumala SE, Messier SE, et al. What is the relationship between gestational age and docosahexaenoic acid (DHA) and arachidonic acid (AA) levels? Prostaglandins Leuko Essent Fatty Acids. 2015;100:5–11.

5 Martin CR, Dasilva DA, Cluette-Brown JE, et al. Decreased postnatal docosahexaenoic acid and arachidonic acid blood levels in premature infants are associated with neonatal morbidities. J Pediatr. 2011;159:743–9.

6 Lofqvist CA, Najm S, Hellgren G, et al. Association of retinopathy of prematurity with low levels of arachidonic acid; a secondary analysis of a randomized clinical trial. JAMA Ophthalmol. 2018;136:271–7.

7 Birch EE, Birch DG, Hoffman DR, Uauy R. Dietary essential fatty acid supply and visual acuity development. Invest Ophthalmol Vis Sci. 1992;33:3242–53.

8 Carlson SE, Werkman SH, Rhodes PG, Tolley EA. Visual acuity development in in healthy preterm infants: effect of marine-oil supplementation. Am J Clin Nutr. 1993;58:35–42.

9 Henriksen C, Haugholt K, Lindgren M, et al. Improved cognitive development among preterm infants attributable to early supplementation of human milk with docosahexaenoic acid and arachidonic acid. Pediatrics. 2008;121:1137–45.

10 Westerberg AC, Schei R, Henriksen C, et al. Attention among very low birth weight infants following early supplementation with docosahexaenoic and arachidonic acid. Acta Paediatr. 2011;100:47–52.

11 Almaas AN, Tamnes CK, Nakstad B, et al. Long-chain polyunsaturated fatty acids and cognition in VLBW infants at 8 years: an RCT. Pediatrics. 2015;135:972–80.

12 Makrides M, Gibson RA, McPhee AJ, et al. Neurodevelopmental outcomes of preterm infants fed high-dose docosahexaenoic acid: a randomised controlled trial. JAMA. 2009;301:175–82.

13 Collins CT, Gibson RA, Anderson PJ, et al. Neurodevelopmental outcomes at 7 years' corrected age in preterm infants who were fed high-dose docosahexaenoic acid to term equivalent: a follow-up of a randomised controlled trial. BMJ Open. 2015;5:e007314. doi:10.1136/bmjopen-2014-007314.

14 Smithers LG, Gibson RA, McPhee A, Makrides M. Higher dose of docosahexaenoic acid in the neonatal period improves visual acuity of preterm infants: results of a randomized controlled trial. Am J Clin Nutr. 2008;88:1049–56.

15 Smithers LG, Collins CT, Simmonds LA, et al. Feeding preterm infants milk with a higher dose of docosahexaenoic acid than that used in current practice does not influence language or behaviour in early childhood: a follow-up of a randomized controlled trial. Am J Clin Nutr. 2010;91:628–34.

16 Molloy CS, Stokes S, Makrides M, et al. Long-term effect of high-dose supplementation with DHA on visual function at school age in children born at <33k wk gestational age: results from a follow-up of a randomized controlled trial. Am J Clin Nutr. 2016;103:268–75.

17 Moltu SJ, Strommen K, Blakstad EW, et al. Enhanced feeding in very-low-birth-weight infants may cause electrolyte disturbances and septicaemia – a randomized, controlled trial. Clin Nutr. 2013;32:207–12.

18 Collins CT, Makrides M, McPhee AJ, et al. Docosahexaenoic acid and bronchopulmonary dysplasia in preterm infants. N Engl J Med. 2017;376:1245–55.

19 Manley BJ, Makrides M, Collins CT, et al. High-dose docosahexaenoic acid supplementation of preterm infants: respiratory and allergy outcomes. Pediatrics. 2011;128.e71–e77.

20 Walsh MC, Yao Q, Gettner P, et al. Impact of a physiologic definition on bronchopulmonary dysplasia rates. Pediatrics. 2004;114:1305–11.

21 Marc I, Piedbouef B, Lacaze-Masmonteil T, et al. Effect of maternal docosahexaenoic acid supplementation on bronchopulmonary dysplasia-free survival in breastfed preterm infants. A randomized clinical trial. JAMA. 2020;342:157–67.

22 Bernabe-Garcia M, Villegas-Silva R, Villavicencio-Torres A, et al. Enteral docosahexaenoic acid and retinopathy of prematurity: a randomized clinical trial. J Parenter Enteral Nutr. 2019;43:874–82.

23 Bernabe-García M, Calder PC, Villegas-Silva R, et al. Efficacy of docosahexaenoic acid for the prevention of necrotising enterocolitis in preterm infants: a randomised clinical trial. Nutrients. 2021;13:648.

24 Hellstrom A, Nilsson AK, Wackernagel D, et al. Effect of enteral lipid supplement on severe retinopathy of prematurity: a randomized clinical trial. JAMA Pediatr. 2021;175:359–67.

25 Makrides M, Collins CT, Gibson RA. Impact of fatty acid status on growth and neurobehavioral development in humans. Matern Child Nutr. 2011;7(Suppl 2):80–88.

26 Hewawasam E, Collins CT, Muhlhausler BS, et al. DHA supplementation in infants born preterm and the effect on attention at 18 months' corrected age: follow-up of a subset of the N3RO randomised controlled trial. Br J Nutr. 2021;125:420–31.

27 Moltu SJ, Blakstad EW, Strommen K, et al. Enhanced feeding and diminished postnatal growth failure in very-low-birth-weight infants. J Pediatr Gastroenterol Nutr. 2014;58:344–51.

28 Martin CR, Zaman MM, Gilkey C, et al. Resolvin D1 and lipoxin A4 improve alveolarization and normalize septal wall thickness in a neonatal murine model of hyperoxia-induced lung disease. PLoS One. 2014;9:e98773.

29 Sapieha P, Stahl A, Chen J, et al. 5-Lipoxenase metabolite 4-HDHA is a mediator of the antiangiogenic effect of omega-3 polyunsaturated fatty acids. Sci Trans Med. 2011;3:69ra12. doi:10.1126/scitranslmed.3001571.

Andrew J. McPhee
SAHMRI Women and Kids
South Australian Health and Medical Research Institute
Level 7, Rieger Building
Women's and Children's Hospital
Adelaide, SA 5006
Australia
andrew.mcphee@sahmri.com

Published online: May 10, 2022

Embleton ND, Haschke F, Bode L (eds): Strategies in Neonatal Care to Promote Optimized Growth and Development: Focus on Low Birth Weight Infants. 96th Nestlé Nutrition Institute Workshop, May 2021. Nestlé Nutr Inst Workshop Ser. Basel, Karger, 2022, vol 96, pp 116–129 (DOI: 10.1159/000519383)

The Potential Role of Nutrition in Modulating the Long-Term Consequences of Early-Life Stress

Hannah G. Juncker[a, b]   Britt J. van Keulen[b, c]
Martijn J.J. Finken[b, c]   Susanne R. de Rooij[d]
Johannes B. van Goudoever[b]   Aniko Korosi[a]

[a]Swammerdam Institute for Life Sciences – Center for Neuroscience, University of Amsterdam, Amsterdam, The Netherlands; [b]Amsterdam UMC, University of Amsterdam, Vrije Universiteit, Emma Children's Hospital, Department of Pediatrics, Amsterdam Reproduction and Development Research Institute, Amsterdam, The Netherlands; [c]Amsterdam UMC, Vrije Universiteit, Emma Children's Hospital, Pediatric Endocrinology, Amsterdam, The Netherlands; [d]Amsterdam UMC, University of Amsterdam, Department of Epidemiology and Data Science, Amsterdam Public Health Institute, Amsterdam, The Netherlands

Abstract

Stress exposure during sensitive developmental periods lastingly affects brain function and cognition and increases vulnerability to psychopathology later in life, as established in various preclinical and clinical studies. Interestingly, similar patterns are seen in children who suffer from perinatal malnutrition. Stress and malnutrition can act closely aligned and stress and nutrition interact. There is emerging evidence that specific nutritional supplementation during various time windows may ameliorate the long-lasting effects of early-life stress, although possible mechanistic insights in this process are sparsely reported. Understanding how stress exposure in early-life influences brain development, and understanding the role of nutrition in this process, is essential for the development of effective (nutritional) therapies to improve long-term health in children exposed to early-life stress. This is especially important in the situation of preterm birth where both stress exposure and malnutrition are common. Here, we will

J.B. van Goudoever and A. Korosi share last authorship.

discuss the programming effects of early-life stress, the possible underlying mechanisms, how nutrients impact on this process, and the promising role of nutrition in modulating (some of) the lasting consequences of early-life stress on brain function and health in adulthood.

The Importance of the Early-Life Environment

The first 1,000 days of life, starting at conception up to approximately 2 years of age, form a critical window in which environmental factors may exert a powerful influence on later health outcomes. This concept is often referred to as the Developmental Origins of Health and Disease [1]. In particular, the first 1,000 days are a period of rapid central nervous system (CNS) development, in which many processes take place, among myelination, neurogenesis, synaptogenesis, cortical layering, and neural circuitry formation throughout various parts in the brain [2]. Environmental factors like stress, but also nutrition, can profoundly influence early brain development [3].

Early-life adversity includes a wide range of experiences, including malnutrition and different forms of stress, among physical stress (e.g., prematurity, prolonged hospital admission, pain) and emotional stress (e.g., parental neglect, physical or emotional abuse). Indeed, increasing evidence from preclinical and clinical studies shows that early-life adversity lastingly affects cognitive functions and increases vulnerability to psychopathology later in life [4–6], although the underlying mechanisms remain elusive.

During fetal and early postnatal life, the brain is the fastest growing organ, thus very high in energy and nutrient demand [7] and therefore very sensitive to malnutrition [8]. There is emerging evidence suggesting that nutrition might play a key role in modulating the effects of early-life stress [9]. Unraveling the important intersection between stress and nutrition in the context of early-life adversity is crucial, especially for premature infants, in which both high levels of stress and malnutrition are common.

First, we will briefly discuss how early-life stress and malnutrition impact on the brain and later life health. Secondly, we will discuss the possible mechanisms involved, with a focus on nutrition. Finally, we will discuss the promising preclinical evidence for nutritional interventions in the prevention of the detrimental effects of early-life stress.

Understanding how stress in early-life influences brain development and understanding how nutrition impacts on this process is essential for the development of effective nutritional therapies to improve long-term health in (preterm) children exposed to early-life stress.

Early-Life Stress and Malnutrition: A Long-Lasting Mark

Over the past decades, an increasing number of studies have identified associations between adverse early-life experiences and a broad range of later-life health outcomes. Indeed, early-life stress is associated with an increased risk of cardiovascular disease, cancer, obesity, and type 2 diabetes mellitus [10]. It is also associated with adverse neurodevelopment and higher rates of mental illnesses like cognitive decline [11], anxiety, and depression in adulthood [10].

The programming effects of early-life stress begin already at conception. Intrauterine life represents one of the most sensitive developmental periods, when the effects of stress are transmitted intergenerationally from a mother to her unborn child as described in many clinical [12, 13] and preclinical [14] studies. For example, high maternal pregnancy-specific anxiety was associated with impaired executive functioning in the children at 7 years of age [15].

Adverse experiences in early life continue to affect an individual's long-term health after birth. Lower maternal affection in early life predicts emotional distress in adulthood [16] and in (pre)term neonates, moderate touch reduced reactivity to stress at adult ages [17]. Animal studies show that adult offspring born to mothers engaging in low levels of licking and grooming behavior increased anxiety-like behavior and physical responses to stress [18, 19]. Interestingly, stroking (simulating of maternal tactile stimuli) reversed these effects [20].

Similar to early-life stress, early-life malnutrition is associated with long-term adverse effects on neurocognitive development, mental health, and behavior. During the sensitive periods of fetal and early neonatal life, even minor nutritional insufficiencies can have adverse long-term effects since they can permanently change brain structure and function [8]. Although all nutrients are necessary for brain growth, key nutrients that support neurodevelopment include macronutrients such as fatty acids and proteins, and micronutrients such as iron, choline, folate, iodine, and vitamins [21]. The effects of undernutrition during pregnancy on adult outcomes have been studied in the Dutch and Chinese famine studies. Individuals exposed to famine prenatally showed poorer visual-motor skills, mental flexibility, and selective attention in a cognitive task in adulthood compared to a control group; furthermore, there were more mental health problems such as anxiety and depression, suggesting a long-lasting negative effect of maternal undernutrition during pregnancy [22, 23].

After birth, the neonate derives its nutrients ideally through breast milk. Differences in breast milk nutrient composition have been associated with child development, for example a positive relation between DHA amounts in breast milk and neurodevelopment of the infants has been shown [24]. More research in this area is needed to better identify the key beneficial components of breast milk for optimal development.

An important condition in which both stress as well as nutritional deficiencies play an important role, is preterm birth. In the last decades, neonatal care has been greatly improved; however, preterm born infants often suffer from long-term psychosocial and neurodevelopmental sequelae including impairments in language skills, memory [25], and executive functions [26]. Preterm infants are separated frequently from their mothers after birth and are exposed to a stressful environment with invasive procedures, interruption of sleep states, shifts in environmental temperature and noise. Also, hits like infections, hypoxic-ischemic insults, and bronchopulmonary dysplasia play a role in long-term detrimental effects. During this period, malnutrition is also playing an important role since administering the right amount of nutrients is still challenging in preterm born infants. One of the most important predicting factors in development after preterm birth is growth rate of the infant, which can be improved significantly by adequate nutrition [27]. Thus, understanding the contribution of the stress, nutrition, and their intersect in the context of preterm care and optimizing this might lead to great advances in long-term health outcomes for preterm born infants.

The precise mechanisms underlying the detrimental and persistent impact of early-life stress on long-term health are currently unknown, even though some structural and functional changes in the brain following early-life stress have been identified. For example, human studies show that early-life stress is associated with a reduction in gray matter volume [28], decreased hippocampal volume [29], and functional and structural changes in cortical/limbic circuits, in particular the prefrontal cortex and the amygdala at different ages later in life [30–32]. Different kinds of abuse seem to be associated with cortical thinning in adulthood [33] and a smaller hippocampus [34, 35]. In line with the human evidence, preclinical models of early-life stress showed impairments of spatial and declarative memory [36] and showed associations with a number of alterations in hippocampal structure, neuronal plasticity [37], and age-dependent changes in adult hippocampal neurogenesis levels [38]. In addition, other experimental animal studies in a wide variety of species demonstrate similar links between early-life stress, brain anatomy/function and mental health throughout life.

Next to early-life stress, perinatal malnutrition shows lasting changes in the brain. For example, in humans, prenatal undernutrition is negatively correlated with total brain volumes at age 68 in men [39], and in animal models, pre- and postnatal iron deficiency is associated with structural and functional changes in the hippocampus [40].

When considering the lasting effects of early-life stress, it is interesting to consider them in an evolutionary perspective. The effects of early-life stress are mostly adaptive responses, to render an individual most fit to the predicted environment. In fact, there is initial evidence that early-life stress, rather than just exerting negative effects, might prepare the offspring to respond optimally under stressful circumstances later in life. This concept is known as the match-mismatch theory [37, 41] and needs further investigation [42].

Considering the observed similarities in neurocognitive, mental, and behavioral outcomes between children exposed to perinatal malnutrition and to early-life stress [43], and the converging mechanisms and interplay between the regulation of stress and the food system, it is interesting to further explore how we can exploit these features. In the next section, we will discuss the possible underlying mechanisms for the long-lasting consequences of early-life stress, and we will discuss how nutrition might be able to impact on these processes.

The Impact of Nutrition on the Programming Pathways of Early-Life Stress

Some of the mechanistic pathways that have been suggested to underlie the programming effects of early-life stress can also be influenced by nutrition; these include among others: (1) the hypothalamic-pituitary-adrenal (HPA) axis; (2) epigenetic mechanisms; (3) oxidative stress; (4) the immune system.

HPA Axis and Glucose Homeostasis
The HPA axis, with glucocorticoids as its end product, is the main neuroendocrine stress system and regulates many body processes, including glucose homeostasis. Early-life stress induces alterations in HPA axis dynamics [44]. Such changes are considered to be instrumental in the link between early-life stress and subsequent brain development. In fact, early-life activation of the HPA axis programs behavioral responses to stress for life, which, in turn, may be a trigger for psychopathology [45]. Studies show that increased cortisol levels in infants are associated with adverse neurodevelopment in childhood [46]. Glucocorticoids are key regulators of glucose homeostasis. During fasting, concentrations of glucocorticoids rise, allowing the release of stored glucose. Moreover, nutritional stimuli, such as the metabolic hormone leptin, have shown to dampen the stress system. Chronic leptin treatment early in life leads to lifelong altered stress-induced HPA axis activity and changes in the hippocampus of rats [47]. In addition, imbalanced perinatal protein and fat intakes have shown to affect HPA axis dynamics [44]. How nutrients interact with glucocorticoids and metabolic hormones is not yet clear and warrants more research.

Epigenetic Mechanisms and Micronutrients

Epigenetic mechanisms determine whether a gene is transcribed or repressed without changing the DNA sequence. In contrast to the genome, the epigenome is dynamic, allowing adaptation to the environment. Over the past few years, a growing body of evidence has implicated epigenetic mechanisms in mediating persistent effects of early-life stress [48]. There is evidence that the epigenome is also affected more globally. For example, whole genome DHA methylation is different between children who were institutionalized and children that were raised by their biological parents [49]. Differences in the amount of perinatal nutrition, including periconceptional nutrition availability [50], are able to cause lasting modifications in DNA methylation and chromatin structure as well [19]. Early-life stress and malnutrition have both been shown to affect acetylation of histones [51]. Thereby, methylation pathways are regulated by dietary factors, both directly but also through provision of methyl groups (vitamin B_{12}, methionine, and choline). Pregnant animals lacking methylation levels in specific gene regions that were fed a methyl-rich diet, produced healthy offspring with high methylation levels in these gene regions [52].

Oxidative Stress and Dietary Antioxidants

Early-life stressful experiences can generate oxidative stress. Oxidative molecules can have an impact on key transcription factors that influence cell signaling pathways involved in proliferation, differentiation, and apoptosis. Therefore, oxidative stress can alter many important reactions that affect development and subsequently influence later life health. The developing brain is particularly sensitive to injury to oxidant molecules [53]. For example, do Prado et al. [54] found oxidative damage in adolescents who were exposed to maltreatment in early life. Antioxidants provided by the diet, such as polyphenol and certain vitamins and minerals, can counteract the detrimental effects of oxidative molecules [55]. Providing adequate nutrition to premature infants can also boost the antioxidant defense mechanisms [56].

Immune System and Fatty Acids

Early-life stress can activate the neuroimmune system via inflammatory pathways within the CNS. Early-life stress induces an immediate immunosuppressive state, but in the long-term, this changes to a proinflammatory state, which triggers secretion of inflammatory molecules [57]. Inflammatory molecules can interact with all of the above-described mechanisms and are known to affect the brain. Moreover, the primary immunocompetent cells of the CNS itself, microglia and astrocytes, are involved in several aspects of brain development and function [58]. Activation of the immune system in early life is associated with (neuro)psychopathologies in adulthood, including cognitive dysfunction [59]. For instance, inflammation during pregnancy is associated with lower IQ in adult men [60]. In addition, pre- and postnatal activation of the immune system have been associated with anxiety-like and depressive-like behavior and cognitive impairments in adulthood [61]. Next to early-life stress, also early-life nutritional insults can affect the neuroimmune system. There are indications for an association between circulating leptin levels and a reduced lymphoproliferative response and proinflammatory cytokine secretion in protein-malnourished infants [62]. Moreover, some specific nutrients have shown to have anti-inflammatory effects, either by directly influencing the immune system or by diminishing oxidative stress, such as fatty acids, polyphenols, and carotenoids [63]. For example, dietary fatty acids have been shown to have a protective effect against many immune-related diseases [64].

Above, a few examples of programming mechanistic pathways for the long-lasting effects of early-life stress, via which nutrients may impact, are mentioned. By no means is this meant to be exhaustive as clearly many other factors and mechanisms have been suggested to play a role in this complex programming of early-life stress such as the microbiome [65].

Importantly, in most studies, the above-described elements (stress and nutrition) and the mechanisms underlying early-life programming are addressed individually. These studies mostly focus on a specific brain region or even cell type. Considering that these mechanisms may have interactions with one another, it is likely that the final effect will be determined by the synergistic action of the different pathways, as depicted in Figure 1. The effects of nutrition on the programming of early-life adversity are complex but may open a window of opportunity for intervention.

The Interplay between Early-Life Factors: Nutritional Interventions

In this section, we will describe some of the evidence for nutritional interventions to mitigate the long-lasting detrimental effects of early-life stress [9], which is largely based on preclinical evidence. For example, supplementation of macronutrients in the form of fat and fatty acids has been shown to prevent the lasting neurocognitive consequences of early-life adversity [66–68]. For example, the offspring of prenatally stressed rats had improved neurocognitive and behavioral outcomes (i.e., protective effect on hippocampus, reduced anxiety, and improved social behavior) if fed a high-fat diet throughout pregnancy and lactation compared with a regular diet [66, 67]. In addition, Yam et al. [68] found that increasing the availability of omega-3 fatty acid in the early-life diet prevents the

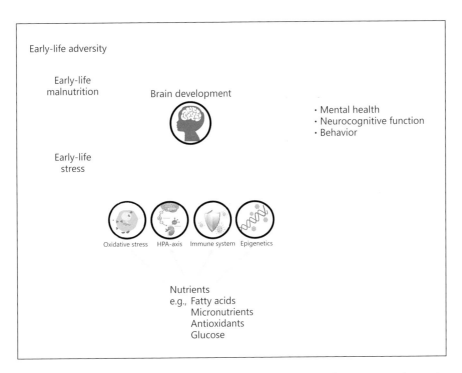

Early-life adversity

Early-life
malnutrition

Brain development

• Mental health
• Neurocognitive function
• Behavior

Early-life
stress

Oxidative stress   HPA-axis   Immune system   Epigenetics

Nutrients
e.g., Fatty acids
Micronutrients
Antioxidants
Glucose

Fig. 1. The long-term consequences of early-life adversity, some of its programming pathways, and the potential role of nutrition in modulating the effects.

early-life stress-induced cognitive impairments associated with a rescue of the early-life stress-induced changes in microglia and neurogenesis. Similarly, early dietary supplementation with essential micronutrients protected against early stress-induced cognitive impairments associated with the blunting of the early-life stress-induced HPA axis hyperactivation [69]. Additionally, choline supplementation to dams during pregnancy and lactation mitigates the effects of in utero stress exposure on adult anxiety-related behaviors [70]. Lastly, Yajima et al. [71] showed that neuronal abnormalities induced by early-life stress in both offspring and mothers may be partially ameliorated by dietary lutein supplementation.

In humans, studies that particularly focus on the effect of nutrition in case of early-life stress are scarce as studying the nutrition-stress interaction in the human setting is difficult, as so many other factors impact on child outcomes. A growing body of evidence found beneficial effects of supplementation with different macro- and micronutrients in developing countries where early-life stress and malnutrition are common. These suggest that several nutrients have a potential beneficial effect on the lasting consequences of early-life adversity, even though stress was not specifically assessed in these studies. An observational study in humans suggests that adequate dietary intakes of the minerals zinc and selenium protect against the adverse effects of prenatal stress exposure on child neurodevelopment [72]. In addition, a low omega-3 to omega-6 ratio in the prenatal diet combined with high prenatal stress resulted in a lower score for orientation and regulation at age 6 months, but only among the children of Afro-American women [73]. Furthermore, prenatal dietary insufficiency of key antioxidant micronutrients was found to exacerbate the effects of prenatal stress on offspring affective behavior [72]. Lastly, Barker et al. [74] demonstrated that a broadly "unhealthy" prenatal and postnatal maternal dietary pattern mediated the adverse effects of prenatal maternal depression on child cognitive function at 8 years of age.

With greater survival rates in premature infants, behavioral and neurocognitive outcomes have become more relevant. Nutritional supplementation studies in preterm infants have shown beneficial effects on neurocognitive development, even after adjusting for confounding factors (i.e., gestational age at delivery, birth weight, and comorbidities). Increased cumulative intakes of energy, protein [75], and lipids [76] have been associated with better developmental outcomes, while the effects of micronutrient supplementation on neurocognitive, mental, and behavioral outcomes in preterm infants, show varying results [77, 78].

In conclusion, early-life nutrition appears to be an appealing candidate for modulating, at least partially, the lasting consequences of early-life stress on adult brain function and health.

Future Perspectives

Early-life stress and perinatal malnutrition lastingly alter brain, behavior, and mental health. This review discussed the rich complexity of the mechanisms underlying its programming effects and emphasizes that still little is known about the exact working and interplay of these pathways.

Over the last years, there has been increased attention to the prevention of the detrimental consequences of stressful experiences in early life. Stress reduction programs for both parents and (preterm) children have been developed [79, 80], and the advantages of family-integrated care are being acknowledged increasingly [81–83].

Specific nutritional support may act as a powerful tool to modify the adverse effects of early-life stress. In animal studies, nutritional supplementations under stressful conditions have shown promising results and seem to be able to modulate the lasting consequences of the early-life stress. In humans, nutritional supplementation in early life has shown beneficial effects; however, up to date, no studies have taken the stress aspects into account within this context. Of note, no studies have been performed to try to counteract or reverse the pathways that lead to the adverse effects of early-life stress in humans. Thereby, the existing evidence is limited by the number of available studies, the heterogeneity of the study designs and the inability to control for confounding variables. Future studies should focus on collecting longitudinal data, unraveling underlying mechanisms in humans, and translating this knowledge into the development of early targeted (nutritional) interventions.

Some of the animal studies show that a nutritional supplement to the lactating dam helps to prevent the lasting effects of early-life stress in her offspring. This raises the question whether breastfeeding also plays a role in the modulation of early-life stress effects in humans. There is initial evidence that maternal stress levels are related to the immunological properties [84] and the microbiome [85] of human milk, but given the above, it could be hypothesized that stress also changes the nutrient composition of breast milk and subsequently the nutrient availability for the infant, which both could be normalized by maternal supplementation. Nutritional supplementation to the mother may be an effective tool in improving the outcome of the offspring. Our ongoing prospective cohort study in the Netherlands is currently investigating the impact of maternal stress on breast milk nutritional composition.

Next to stress reduction programs like family integrated care, the development of nutritional interventions to reduce the adverse effects of early-life stress is promising as nutritional interventions are relatively safe, inexpensive, and easy to implement. To be able to develop nutritional interventions for humans (pregnant/lactating mothers and infant), understanding the timing of critical developmental periods and the mechanisms and interactions involved in the programming of early-life adversity is crucial. Combining these factors may significantly improve short- and long-term child health with subsequently economic and societal benefits in children exposed to early-life stress.

Conclusion

Stress and malnutrition in early life have a major impact on the well-being of the infant, which exerts its effect into adulthood. Stress-reducing programs and targeted nutritional interventions for both mother and child may alleviate the long-term consequences of early-life adversity.

Conflicts of Interest Statement

J.B.G. is founder and director of the Dutch National Human Milk Bank and member of the National Health Council. The other authors have no conflict of interest to declare.

References

1 Gluckman PD, Hanson MA. Living with the past: evolution, development, and patterns of disease. Science. 2004 Sep;305(5691):1733–6.
2 Tau GZ, Peterson BS. Normal development of brain circuits. Neuropsychopharmacology. 2010 Jan;35(1):147–68.
3 Lebel C, Deoni S. The development of brain white matter microstructure. Neuroimage. 2018 Nov;182:207–218.
4 Loman MM, Gunnar MR. Early experience and the development of stress reactivity and regulation in children. Neurosci Biobehav Rev. 2010 May;34(6):867–76.
5 Pesonen AK, et al. Cognitive ability and decline after early life stress exposure. Neurobiol Aging. 2013 Jun;34(6):1674–9.
6 Alastalo H, et al. Early life stress and physical and psychosocial functioning in late adulthood. PLoS One. 2013 Jul;8(7):e69011.
7 Bourre JM. Effects of nutrients (in food) on the structure and function of the nervous system: Update on dietary requirements for brain. Part 1: Micronutrients. J Nutr Health Aging. Sep-Oct 2006;10(5):377–85.
8 Prado EL, Dewey KG. Nutrition and brain development in early life. Nutr Rev. 2014 Apr;72(4):267–84.
9 Lucassen PJ, Naninck EFG, van Goudoever JB, et al. Perinatal programming of adult hippocampal structure and function; emerging roles of stress, nutrition and epigenetics. Trends Neurosci. 2013 Nov;36(11):621–31.
10 Norman RE, Byambaa M, De R, Butchart A, Scott J, Vos T. The long-term health consequences of child physical abuse, emotional abuse, and neglect: a systematic review and meta-analysis. PLoS Med. 2012;9(11):e1001349.
11 Ritchie K, et al. Adverse childhood environment and late-life cognitive functioning. Int J Geriatr Psychiatry. 2011 May;26(5):503–10.
12 Hughes K, et al. The effect of multiple adverse childhood experiences on health: a systematic review and meta-analysis. Lancet Public Health. 2017 Aug;2(8):e356–e366.
13 Bellis MA, Hughes K, Ford K, et al. Life course health consequences and associated annual costs of adverse childhood experiences across Europe and North America: a systematic review and meta-analysis. Lancet Public Health. 2019 Oct;4(10):e517–e528.

14 Chan JC, Nugent BM, Bale TL. Parental advisory: maternal and paternal stress can impact offspring neurodevelopment. Biol Psychiatry. 2018 May;83(10):886–894.
15 Buss C, Davis EP, Hobel CJ, Sandman CA. Maternal pregnancy-specific anxiety is associated with child executive function at 69 years age. Stress. 2011 Nov;14(6):665–76.
16 Maselko J, Kubzansky L, Lipsitt L, Buka SL. Mother's affection at 8 months predicts emotional distress in adulthood. J Epidemiol Community Health. 2011 Jul;65(7):621–5.
17 Feldman R, Singer M, Zagoory O. Touch attenuates infants' physiological reactivity to stress. Dev Sci. 2010 Mar;13(2):271–8.
18 van Hasselt FN, et al. Adult hippocampal glucocorticoid receptor expression and dentate synaptic plasticity correlate with maternal care received by individuals early in life. Hippocampus. 2012 Feb;22(2):255–66.
19 Weaver ICG, et al. Epigenetic programming by maternal behavior. Nat Neurosci. 2004 Aug;7(8):847–54.
20 Chatterjee D, Chatterjee-Chakraborty M, Rees S, et al. Maternal isolation alters the expression of neural proteins during development: "Stroking" stimulation reverses these effects. Brain Res. 2007 Jul;1158:11–27.
21 Georgieff MK, Brunette KE, Tran PV. Early life nutrition and neural plasticity. Dev Psychopathol. 2015 May;27(2):411–23.
22 De Rooij SR, Wouters H, Yonker JE, et al. Prenatal undernutrition and cognitive function in late adulthood. Proc Natl Acad Sci USA. 2010 Sep;107(39):16881–6.
23 Yehuda R, Engel SM, Brand SR, et al. Transgenerational effects of posttraumatic stress disorder in babies of mothers exposed to the World Trade Center attacks during pregnancy. J Clin Endocrinol Metab. 2005 Jul;90(7):4115–8.
24 Campoy C, Escolano-Margarit V, Anjos T, et al. Omega 3 fatty acids on child growth, visual acuity and neurodevelopment. Br J Nutr. 2012 Jun;107 Suppl 2:S85–106.
25 Nosarti C, Murray RM, Hack M. Neurodevelopmental Outcomes of Preterm Birth: From Childhood to Adult Life. Cambridge: Cambridge University Press; 2010.

26 Twilhaar ES, Wade RM, De Kieviet JF, et al. Cognitive outcomes of children born extremely or very preterm since the 1990s and associated risk factors: A meta-analysis and meta-regression. JAMA Pediatr. 2018 Apr;172(4):361–367.

27 Koletzko B, Poindexter B, Uauy R, editors. Nutritional Care of Preterm Infants. Basel: Karger; 2014.

28 Sandman CA, Buss C, Head K, Davis EP. Fetal exposure to maternal depressive symptoms is associated with cortical thickness in late childhood. Biol Psychiatry. 2015 Feb;77(4):324–34.

29 Frodl T, Reinhold E, Koutsouleris N, et al. Interaction of childhood stress with hippocampus and prefrontal cortex volume reduction in major depression. J Psychiatr Res. 2010 Oct;44(13):799–807.

30 De Brito SA, et al. Reduced orbitofrontal and temporal grey matter in a community sample of maltreated children. J Child Psychol Psychiatry Allied Discip. 2013 Jan;54(1):105–12.

31 Hanson JL, et al. Early stress is associated with alterations in the orbitofrontal cortex: A tensor-based morphometry investigation of brain structure and behavioral risk. J Neurosci. 2010 Jun;30(22):7466–72.

32 Dannlowski U, et al. Limbic scars: Long-term consequences of childhood maltreatment revealed by functional and structural magnetic resonance imaging. Biol Psychiatry. 2012 Feb;71(4):286–93.

33 Heim CM, Mayberg HS, Mletzko T, et al. Decreased cortical representation of genital somatosensory field after childhood sexual abuse. Am J Psychiatry. 2013 Jun;170(6):616–23.

34 Hanson JL, et al. Behavioral problems after early life stress: contributions of the hippocampus and amygdala. Biol Psychiatry. 2015 Feb;77(4):314–23.

35 Teicher MH, Samson JA. Annual research review: enduring neurobiological effects of childhood abuse and neglect. J Child Psychol Psychiatry. 2016 Mar;57(3):241–66.

36 Rice CJ, Sandman CA, Lenjavi MR, Baram TZ. A novel mouse model for acute and long-lasting consequences of early life stress. Endocrinology. 2008 Oct;149(10):4892–900.

37 Oomen CA, et al. Severe early life stress hampers spatial learning and neurogenesis, but improves hippocampal synaptic plasticity and emotional learning under high-stress conditions in adulthood. J Neurosci. 2010 May;30(19):6635–45.

38 Huot RL, Plotsky PM, Lenox RH, McNamara RK. Neonatal maternal separation reduces hippocampal mossy fiber density in adult Long Evans rats. Brain Res. 2002 Sep;950(1-2):52–63.

39 De Rooij SR, et al. Prenatal famine exposure has sex-specific effects on brain size. Brain. 2016 Aug;139(Pt 8):2136–42.

40 Tran PV, Fretham SJB, Wobken J, et al. Gestational-neonatal iron deficiency suppresses and iron treatment reactivates IGF signaling in developing rat hippocampus. Am J Physiol Endocrinol Metab. 2012 Feb;302(3):E316–24.

41 Nederhof E, Schmidt MV. Mismatch or cumulative stress: toward an integrated hypothesis of programming effects. Physiol Behav. 2012 Jul;106(5):691–700.

42 Frankenhuis WE, Young ES, Ellis BJ. The hidden talents approach: theoretical and methodological challenges. Trends Cogn Sci. 2020 Jul;24(7):569–581.

43 Lindsay KL, Buss C, Wadhwa PD, Entringer S. The interplay between maternal nutrition and stress during pregnancy: issues and considerations. Ann Nutr Metab. 2017;70(3):191–200.

44 Yam KY, Naninck EFG, Schmidt MV, Lucassen PJ, Korosi A. Early-life adversity programs emotional functions and the neuroendocrine stress system: the contribution of nutrition, metabolic hormones and epigenetic mechanisms. Stress. 2015;18(3):328–42.

45 Abe H, et al. Prenatal psychological stress causes higher emotionality, depression-like behavior, and elevated activity in the hypothalamo-pituitary-adrenal axis. Neurosci Res. 2007 Oct;59(2):145–51.

46 Herbert J, et al. Do corticosteroids damage the brain? J Neuroendocrinol. 2006 Jun;18(6):393–411.

47 Proulx K. High neonatal leptin exposure enhances brain GR expression and feedback efficacy on the adrenocortical axis of developing rats. Endocrinology. 2001 Nov;142(11):4607–16.

48 Szyf M. The epigenetics of perinatal stress. Dialogues Clin Neurosci. 2019 Dec;21(4):369–378.

49 Naumova OY, Lee M, Koposov R, et al. Differential patterns of whole-genome DNA methylation in institutionalized children and children raised by their biological parents. Dev Psychopathol. 2012 Feb;24(1):143–55.

50 Dominguez-Salas P, et al. Maternal nutrition at conception modulates DNA methylation of human metastable epialleles. Nat Commun. 2014 Apr;5:3746.

51 Levine A, Worrell TR, Ziminsky R, Schmauss C. Early life stress triggers sustained changes in histone deacetylase expression and histone H4 modifications that alter responsiveness to adolescent antidepressant treatment. Neurobiol Dis. 2012 Jan;45(1):488–98.

52 Stevens AJ, Rucklidge JJ, Kennedy MA. Epigenetics, nutrition and mental health. Is there a relationship? Nutr Neurosci. 2018 Nov;21(9):602–613.

53 Dennery PA. Oxidative stress in development: nature or nurture? Free Radic Biol Med. 2010 Oct;49(7):1147–51.

54 do Prado CH, et al. The impact of childhood maltreatment on redox state: Relationship with oxidative damage and antioxidant defenses in adolescents with no psychiatric disorder. Neurosci Lett. 2016 Mar;617:173-7.

55 Bjørklund G, Chirumbolo S. Role of oxidative stress and antioxidants in daily nutrition and human health. Nutrition. 2017 Jan;33:311–321.

56 Te Braake FWJ, et al. Glutathione synthesis rates after amino acid administration directly after birth in preterm infants. Am J Clin Nutr. 2008 Aug;88(2):333–9.

57 Hoeijmakers L, Lucassen PJ, Korosi A. The interplay of early-life stress, nutrition, and immune activation programs adult hippocampal structure and function. Front Mol Neurosci. 2015 Jan;7:103.

58 Bilbo SD, Schwarz JM. The immune system and developmental programming of brain and behavior. Front Neuroendocrinol. 2012 Aug;33(3):267–86.

59 O'Connor TG, Moynihan JA, Caserta MT. Annual research review: the neuroinflammation hypothesis for stress and psychopathology in children – developmental psychoneuroimmunology. J Child Psychol Psychiatry. 2014 Jun;55(6):615–31.

60 Eriksen W, Sundet JM, Tambs K. Register data suggest lower intelligence in men born the year after flu pandemic. Ann Neurol. 2009 Sep;66(3):284–9.

61 Dinel AL, et al. Inflammation early in life is a vulnerability factor for emotional behavior at adolescence and for lipopolysaccharide-induced spatial memory and neurogenesis alteration at adulthood. J Neuroinflammation. 2014 Sep;11:155.

62 Palacio A, Lopez M, Perez-Bravo F, et al. Leptin levels are associated with immune response in malnourished infants. J Clin Endocrinol Metab. 2002 Jul;87(7):3040–6.

63 Tan BL, Norhaizan ME, Liew WPP. Nutrients and oxidative stress: friend or foe? Oxid Med Cell Longev. 2018 Jan;2018:9719584.

64 Radzikowska U, et al. The influence of dietary fatty acids on immune responses. Nutrients. 2019 Dec;11(12):2990.

65 Osadchiy V, Martin CR, Mayer EA. The gut-brain axis and the microbiome: mechanisms and clinical implications. Clin Gastroenterol Hepatol. 2019 Jan;17(2):322–332.

66 Huang CF, et al. Effect of prenatal exposure to LPS combined with pre- and post-natal high-fat diet on hippocampus in rat offspring. Neuroscience. 2015 Feb;286:364–70.

67 Rincel M, et al. Maternal high-fat diet prevents developmental programming by early-life stress. Transl Psychiatry. 2016 Nov;6(11):e966.

68 Yam KY, et al. Increasing availability of ω-3 fatty acid in the early-life diet prevents the early-life stress-induced cognitive impairments without affecting metabolic alterations. FASEB J. 2019 Apr;33(4):5729–5740.

69 Naninck EFG, et al. Early micronutrient supplementation protects against early stress-induced cognitive impairments. FASEB J. 2017 Feb;31(2):505–518.

70 Schulz KM, et al. Dietary choline supplementation to dams during pregnancy and lactation mitigates the effects of in utero stress exposure on adult anxiety-related behaviors. Behav Brain Res. 2014 Jul;268:104–10.

71 Yajima M, Matsumoto M, Harada M, Hara H, Yajima T. Effects of constant light during perinatal periods on the behavioral and neuronal development of mice with or without dietary lutein. Biomed Res. 2013 Aug;34(4):197–204.

72 Lipton LR, et al. Associations among prenatal stress, maternal antioxidant intakes in pregnancy, and child temperament at age 30 months. J Dev Orig Health Dis. 2017 Dec;8(6):638–648.

73 Brunst KJ, et al. Effects of prenatal social stress and maternal dietary fatty acid ratio on infant temperament: does race matter? Epidemiology (Sunnyvale). 2014;4(4):1000167.

74 Barker ED, Kirkham N, Ng J, Jensen SKG. Prenatal maternal depression symptoms and nutrition, and child cognitive function. Br J Psychiatry. 2013 Dec;203(6):417–21.

75 Stephens BE, et al. First-week protein and energy intakes are associated with 18-month developmental outcomes in extremely low birth weight infants. Pediatrics. 2009 May;123(5):1337–43.

76 Eleni dit Trolli S, Kermorvant-Duchemin E, Huon C, et al. Early lipid supply and neurological development at one year in very low birth weight (VLBW) preterm infants. Early Hum Dev. 2012 Mar;88 Suppl 1:S25–9.

77 Ambalavanan N, et al. Vitamin A supplementation for extremely low birth weight infants: outcome at 18 to 22 months. Pediatrics. 2005 Mar;115(3):e249–54.

78 Jin HX, Wang RS, Chen SJ, et al. Early and late iron supplementation for low birth weight infants: a meta-analysis. Ital J Pediatr. 2015 Mar;41:16.

79 Urizar GG, Yim IS, Rodriguez A, Schetter CD. The SMART Moms Program: a randomized trial of the impact of stress management on perceived stress and cortisol in low-income pregnant women. Psychoneuroendocrinology. 2019 Jun;104:174–184.

80 Lenz B, et al. Mindfulness-based stress reduction in pregnancy: an app-based programme to improve the health of mothers and children (MINDFUL/PMI Study). Geburtshilfe Frauenheilkd. 2018 Dec;78(12):1283–1291.

81 Franck LS, O'Brien K. The evolution of family-centered care: from supporting parent-delivered interventions to a model of family integrated care. Birth Defects Res. 2019 Sep;111(15):1044–1059.

82 van Veenendaal NR, et al. Hospitalising preterm infants in single family rooms versus open bay units: a systematic review and meta-analysis. Lancet Child Adolesc Heal. 2019 Mar;3(3):147–157.

83 van Veenendaal NR, et al. Family integrated care in single family rooms for preterm infants and late-onset sepsis: a retrospective study and mediation analysis. Pediatr Res. 2020 Oct;88(4):593–600.

84 Moirasgenti M, Doulougeri K, Panagopoulou E, Theodoridis T. Psychological stress reduces the immunological benefits of breast milk. Stress Health. 2019 Dec;35(5):681–685.

85 Browne PD, et al. Human milk microbiome and maternal postnatal psychosocial distress. Front Microbiol. 2019 Oct;10:2333.

Johannes B. van Goudoever
Vrije Universiteit, Department of Pediatrics
Emma Children's Hospital
Amsterdam UMC, University of Amsterdam
Meibergdreef 9
NL–1100 DD Amsterdam
h.vangoudoever@amsterdamumc.nl

Published online: May 10, 2022

Embleton ND, Haschke F, Bode L (eds): Strategies in Neonatal Care to Promote Optimized Growth and Development: Focus on Low Birth Weight Infants. 96th Nestlé Nutrition Institute Workshop, May 2021. Nestlé Nutr Inst Workshop Ser. Basel, Karger, 2022, vol 96, pp 130–137 (DOI: 10.1159/000519393)

Micronutrient Intakes and Health Outcomes in Preterm Infants

Magnus Domellöf

Department of Clinical Sciences, Pediatrics, Umeå University, Umeå, Sweden

Abstract

Deficiency or excess of specific micronutrients is common in preterm infants and can have many effects on health outcomes, ranging from life-threatening electrolyte disturbances to long-term effects on growth, brain development, bone health, and the risk of retinopathy of prematurity (ROP). Iron supplementation of low birth weight infants reduces the risk of behavioral problems. However, due to the risk of adverse effects, iron supplementation of very preterm infants in the NICU should be individualized, considering birth weight, postnatal age, diet, and serum ferritin concentrations. Sodium intakes should be minimized during the first 3 days of life in very preterm infants to avoid hypernatremia. However, after 4 days of age, sodium supplements can reduce hyponatremia and improve growth. Adequate parenteral and enteral calcium and phosphorus intakes are crucial for the prevention of osteopenia of prematurity. Screening of serum phosphate concentrations is useful. Deficiencies of docosahexaenoic acid (DHA) and arachidonic acid (AA) are frequently observed in extremely preterm infants. A recent Swedish study suggests that combined DHA and AA supplementation may reduce the risk of severe ROP. When prescribing enteral and parenteral nutrition for preterm infants, it is important to consider micronutrients. Many preterm infants will need different micronutrient supplements. © 2022 S. Karger AG, Basel

Micronutrients can be defined as all nutrients except the macronutrients (protein, fat, and carbohydrates). This definition includes all minerals, vitamins, and trace elements, for which recommended daily intakes in preterm infants are typically given in mg or µg rather than grams per kg. Essential fatty acids such as long-chain polyunsaturated fatty acids are often also included in the definition of micronutrients. Micronutrients do not contribute to any significant extent to the energy intake but are essential for a vast array of specific functions in the body.

Deficient or excessive intakes of micronutrients are common in preterm infants [1]. Deficiency or excess of a specific micronutrient can have a drastic health impact in preterm infants, such as a massive intracranial hemorrhage caused by vitamin K deficiency, life-threatening arrythmias caused by hyperkalemia or a femoral fracture due to calcium and phosphate deficiency. However, in most cases, micronutrients have more subtle, but still extremely important health effects on, e.g., growth, brain development, bone health, and the risk of retinopathy of prematurity (ROP), see Figure 1.

We have used iron as a model nutrient in our studies of the effects of early micronutrient intakes on long-term health. Iron is essential for heme synthesis, oxygen transport, and many enzyme functions. The capacity of iron to switch between its two oxidation states Fe^{2+} (ferrous) and Fe^{3+} (ferric) underlies its essential role in oxygen transport and electron transfer reactions. Preterm and low birth weight infants are at high risk of iron deficiency due to low iron stores at birth, high iron requirements due to rapid growth and iron losses due to frequent blood samplings during neonatal intensive care. Iron deficiency (ID) leads to anemia and may have adverse effects on brain development. Iron is essential for neurogenesis and the differentiation of brain cells during the third trimester, which is a sensitive period of brain growth and development. In animal models, a clear causal relationship has been demonstrated between ID in infancy and impaired brain development and function, an effect which may be irreversible. Several domains of brain function have been shown in animal models to be affected by ID, including myelination, neurotransmitter synthesis and function, energy metabolism, and neuronal growth and dendrite formation [2].

We randomized 285 otherwise healthy infants with marginally low birth weight (2,000–2,500 g) to receive 0, 1, or 2 mg/kg/day of iron supplements from 6 weeks of age until 6 months of age [3]. About 50% of these infants were preterm, the rest term, small for gestational age. Iron supplementation significantly reduced iron deficiency and iron deficiency anemia at 6 months: in the placebo group, 36% of the infants had iron deficiency, and 10% had iron deficiency anemia, while the corresponding proportions were 4 and 0% in the 2 mg iron group [3]. At 3 years of age, the previously iron supplemented infants had significantly lower risk of behavioral problems, OR 0.24 (95% CI 0.07–0.84), and this effect remained at 7 years of

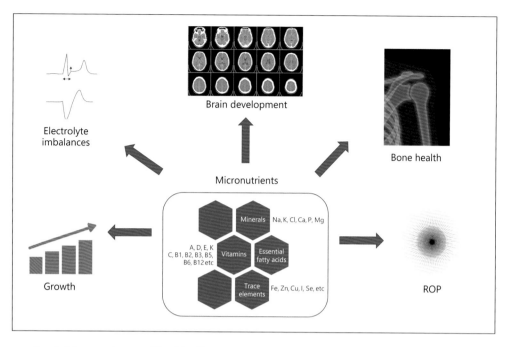

Fig. 1. Micronutrients and health effects in preterm infants.

age [4, 5]. Interestingly, the effect on behavioral problems at 7 years was mainly seen in externalizing behavior. This study together with other evidence is the basis of the current recommendation that all low birth weight infants should receive iron supplements during the first 6 months of life [6].

However, humans have no mechanism for iron excretion; iron is a highly reactive pro-oxidant and an essential nutrient for many pathogens. Thus, excessive iron supplements can have adverse effects, e.g. infections, diarrhea, poor growth, and even poor neurodevelopment [7]. It has recently been shown that iron supplements can cause dysbiosis of the gut microbiome, which may be a mechanism for some of these adverse effects. In a study of 72 healthy, iron-sufficient, non-anemic 6-month-old infants randomized to iron drops (6.6 mg/day), high-iron formula (6.6 mg/day) or low-iron formula (1.3 mg/day) during 45 days, infants receiving iron drops had less lactobacillus and streptococcus and more clostridium and bacteroides species in the gut microbiome [8]. Preterm infants receiving multiple blood transfusions are also at risk of iron overload, and local practice regarding blood sampling, blood transfusions and erythropoietin treatment greatly influences iron requirements in very low birth weight infants [9]. For these reasons, it is important to individualize iron supplements for very preterm infants during the stay at the neonatal intensive care unit (NICU), considering birth weight, postnatal age, diet, and serum ferritin concentrations [7].

Zinc is a micronutrient which is essential for growth, immune defense, and wound healing. Unlike iron, there are no toxicity problems – the main concern with higher zinc intakes is an increased copper requirement due to competition at the intestinal absorption stage [10]. Traditional fetal accretion calculations have been based on preterm infants with weights between 1,500 and 2,000 g, but the theoretical requirements are higher for infants <1,500 g. A recent Cochrane meta-analysis concludes that zinc supplements for preterm infants may decrease mortality and probably improves weight gain and linear growth [11]. However, the included studies used quite different doses of zinc. In conclusion, zinc requirements in very low birth weight infants are probably higher than previously believed, likely about 2–3 mg/kg/day.

Sodium is the principal cation in extracellular fluid and its concentration influences intravascular and interstitial volumes and blood pressure. Sodium is important for growth but also plays roles in such diverse processes as bone mineralization, nerve conduction, and nitrogen retention. Preterm infants are at risk of both hypernatremia and hyponatremia during the NICU stay. A slight increase in plasma sodium during the first 3 days of life is normal in newborns and reflects the postnatal weight loss and fluid loss from the extracellular compartment. Hypernatremia can be more severe in extremely preterm infants and typically reaches a peak at 3 days of age [12]. It is therefore recommended to minimize sodium intakes during the first 3 days of life in very preterm infants. However, after 4 days of age, hyponatremia becomes more common and iron requirements are high (3–8 mmol/kg/day) during the rest of the NICU stay. The reason for this is immature sodium reabsorption in the renal tubuli leading to sodium losses in the urine. Sodium supplements are thus frequently needed after the first few days of life in very preterm infants and have been shown to improve growth [13].

Calcium, phosphorus, magnesium, and vitamin D are some micronutrients which are essential for bone growth and development. Osteopenia or metabolic bone disease of prematurity is usually caused by deficiencies in calcium and phosphorus, since these two minerals are especially difficult to deliver in sufficient quantities both in parenteral and enteral nutrition due to their tendency for precipitation. Osteopenia is associated with dolichocephalic head flattening of preterm infants, and severe osteopenia leads to fractures. Along with improved nutrition, the incidence of rickets in infants with birth weight <1,000 g has decreased from approximately 50% in the 1980s to about 15% [14]. However, severe cases with fractures are still occasionally seen today in NICUs, and infants on long-term parenteral nutrition are at especially high risk. In order to prevent osteopenia, it is important to provide adequate amounts of calcium, phosphorus, and vitamin D to all preterm infants. In addition, screening tests are recommended in order to optimize calcium and phosphorus intakes and to discover early signs of osteopenia [15]. Screening may involve serum measurements of phosphate, alkaline phosphatase, and parathyroid hormone, or concentrations of calcium and phosphate in urine. Even though a low serum phosphate concentration is a hallmark of osteopenia after the first few weeks of life in preterm infants, it is important to note that osteopenic infants usually have normal or high serum calcium concentrations.

In addition to the late hypophosphatemia of osteopenia, early hypophosphatemia is commonly observed in very low birth weight infants during the first week of life. Some of these infants have severe hypophosphatemia (<1.0 mmol/L), which can lead to life-threatening cardiac arrythmias and may increase the risk of sepsis [16]. The mechanism behind early hypophosphatemia is not phosphorus deficiency but rather a temporary shift of electrolytes between body fluid compartments, similar to refeeding syndrome [17]. Amino acids from parenteral nutrition are transported into cells together with phosphorus and potassium, depleting the extracellular compartment of these two cations. The resulting hypophosphatemia causes phosphorus to be released from bone tissue, leading to an increase in serum calcium. Thus, this condition is characterized not only by hypophosphatemia but also hypokalemia and hypercalcemia.

Linoleic acid and alpha linolenic acid are the essential fatty acids in the omega 6 and omega 3 series, respectively. These are converted in the liver by the delta 6 desaturase to form arachidonic acid (AA) and eicosapentaenoic acid, which in turn is converted to docosahexaenoic acid (DHA). Even though late or moderately preterm infants have similar delta 6 desaturase activity as term infants [18], very preterm infants are believed to have an immature delta 6 desaturase activity, and DHA and AA, and very low levels of serum DHA and AA have been observed from 7 days of age in extremely preterm infants, even when they receive modern parenteral nutrition solutions, which provide insufficient amounts of DHA and AA [19]. Since long-chain polyunsaturated fatty acids are essential for normal brain and eye development, it is important to ensure an adequate intake of DHA and AA in the diet of very preterm infants. Notably, these fatty acids are present in breast milk, but the concentrations are highly dependent on the maternal diet, which are commonly lacking in fish and seafood. In an Australian study, 1,273 preterm infants born before 29 gestational weeks were randomized to DHA (60 mg/kg/day) or placebo [20]. Since low DHA levels have been associated with BPD, the primary outcome in this study was BPD. Unexpectedly, the study instead showed an increased risk of BPD (aOR 1.13, 95% CI 1.02–1.25) as well as increased risk of BPD or death (aOR 1.11, 95% CI 1.00–1.23) in the DHA group. Notably, the intervention did not include AA.

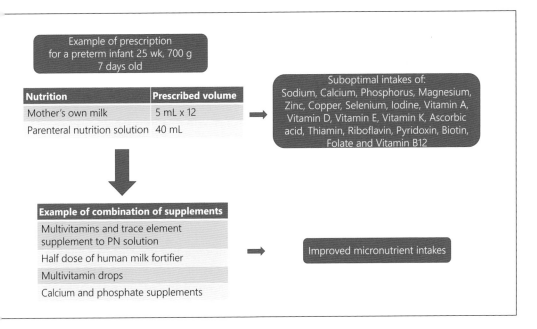

Fig. 2. Examples of micronutrient supplements for preterm infants.

In a recent Swedish study, 101 extremely preterm infants born <28 weeks of gestation were randomized to receive supplements with DHA (50 mg/kg/day) and AA (100 mg/kg/day) or placebo from <3 days until term age, the primary outcome being severe ROP [21]. Interestingly, the incidence of severe ROP was significantly reduced with a risk ratio of 0.50 (95% CI 0.28–0.91, $p = 0.02$). This suggests that extremely preterm infants may benefit from combined DHA and AA supplementation. The safety and efficacy of this intervention is currently being evaluated in a Norwegian randomized, controlled trial involving 120 preterm infants born before 29 weeks of gestation [22]. The primary outcome of that trial is brain maturation as assessed by magnetic resonance imaging at term age, which hopefully also will give more insight on the effects of DHA and AA supplements on brain development in preterm infants.

Even though the examples given above only cover a few micronutrients, they highlight the importance of micronutrients for short- and long-term health outcomes in preterm infants. When prescribing enteral and parenteral nutrition for preterm infants, it is important to consider not only macronutrients but also the micronutrients. Parenteral nutrition solutions need to have an appropriate micronutrient balance to cover requirements without causing excessive intakes of some micronutrients, which may have adverse effects. Likewise, human milk fortifiers and preterm formulas need to have an appropriate micronutrient composition. Especially challenging clinical situations are preterm infants who are on a combination of enteral and parenteral nutrition, and fully breast milk-fed infants who do not receive full-dose human milk fortifier. Many preterm infants will need additional micronutrient supplements, which may involve several separate supplements of vitamins, different minerals, and trace elements (see Fig. 2).

Parenteral micronutrient requirements for preterm infants are published in the ESGPHAN/ESPEN/ESPR/CSPEN guidelines on pediatric parenteral nutrition from 2018 [23]. Enteral micronutrient requirements for preterm infants are included in the ESPGHAN recommendations from 2010 [24], but these guidelines are currently being updated, with estimated publication in late 2021 or early 2022. A difficulty when prescribing a combination of enteral and parenteral nutrition is that it is not possible to add the micronutrient intakes from these two sources (which is commonly done for macronutrients) since the intestinal absorption of different micronutrients ranges between 8 and 100% with many micronutrients having a bioavailability of around 50% or lower [1]. Modern software tools allow calculation of micronutrient intakes also for preterm infants who receive a combination of enteral and parenteral nutrition as well as different supplements and fortifiers, which facilitates correct prescriptions and improves micronutrient intakes [25].

Our knowledge on micronutrient requirements in preterm infants is still far from complete, even though several of the micronutrients are targets of active research. Results of future research will give even better data upon which to base recommendations for improved short- and long-term health in preterm infants.

Conflict of Interest Statement

Magnus Domellöf has received honoraria or consultation/speaker fees from Abbvie AB, Arla Foods Ingredients, Baxter AB, Biostime Institute of Nutrition and Care, Chiesi Pharma AB, Danone Nutricia, Fresenius Kabi Sweden, Mead Johnson, Nestec Ltd. (Nestlé), Prolacta Bioscience and Semper AB, as well as grants/research supports from Baxter AB and Prolacta Bioscience.

References

1 Sjostrom ES, Ohlund I, Ahlsson F, Domellof M. Intakes of micronutrients are associated with early growth in extremely preterm infants. J Pediatr Gastroenterol Nutr. 2016;62(6):885–92.

2 Beard J. Recent evidence from human and animal studies regarding iron status and infant development. J Nutr. 2007;137(2):524S–30S.

3 Berglund S, Westrup B, Domellof M. Iron supplements reduce the risk of iron deficiency anemia in marginally low birth weight infants. Pediatrics. 2010;126(4):e874–83.

4 Berglund SK, Westrup B, Hägglöf B, et al. Effects of iron supplementation of LBW infants on cognition and behavior at 3 years. Pediatrics. 2013;131(1):47–55.

5   Berglund SK, Chmielewska A, Starnberg J, et al. Effects of iron supplementation of low-birth-weight infants on cognition and behavior at 7 years: a randomized controlled trial. Pediatr Res. 2018;83(1–1):111–8.

6   Domellof M, Braegger C, Campoy C, et al. Iron requirements of infants and toddlers. J Pediatr Gastroenterol Nutr. 2014;58(1):119–29.

7   Domellof M. Meeting the iron needs of low and very low birth weight infants. Ann Nutr Metab. 2017;71(Suppl 3):16–23.

8   Simonyte Sjodin K, Domellof M, Lagerqvist C, et al. Administration of ferrous sulfate drops has significant effects on the gut microbiota of iron-sufficient infants: a randomised controlled study. Gut. 2019;68(11):2095–7.

9   Alm S, Stoltz Sjostrom E, Nilsson Sommar J, Domellof M. Erythrocyte transfusions increased the risk of elevated serum ferritin in very low birthweight infants and were associated with altered longitudinal growth. Acta Paediatr. 2020;109(7):1354–60.

10 Griffin IJ, Domellof M, Bhatia J, et al. Zinc and copper requirements in preterm infants: an examination of the current literature. Early Hum Dev. 2013;89(Suppl 2):S29–34.

11 Staub E, Evers K, Askie LM. Enteral zinc supplementation for prevention of morbidity and mortality in preterm neonates. Cochrane Database Syst Rev. 2021;3:CD012797.

12 Spath C, Sjostrom ES, Ahlsson F, et al. Sodium supply influences plasma sodium concentration and the risks of hyper- and hyponatremia in extremely preterm infants. Pediatr Res. 2017;81(3):455–60.

13 Isemann B, Mueller EW, Narendran V, Akinbi H. Impact of early sodium supplementation on hyponatremia and growth in premature infants: a randomized controlled trial. JPEN J Parenter Enteral Nutr. 2016;40(3):342–9.

14 Chinoy A, Mughal MZ, Padidela R. Metabolic bone disease of prematurity: causes, recognition, prevention, treatment and long-term consequences. Arch Dis Child Fetal Neonatal Ed. 2019;104(5):F560–F6.

15 Abrams SA, Committee on Nutrition. Calcium and vitamin D requirements of enterally fed preterm infants. Pediatrics. 2013;131(5):e1676–83.

16 Moltu SJ, Strommen K, Blakstad EW, et al. Enhanced feeding in very-low-birth-weight infants may cause electrolyte disturbances and septicemia – a randomized, controlled trial. Clin Nutr. 2013;32(2):207–12.

17 Bonsante F, Iacobelli S, Latorre G, et al. Initial amino acid intake influences phosphorus and calcium homeostasis in preterm infants – it is time to change the composition of the early parenteral nutrition. PLoS One. 2013;8(8):e72880.

18 Nagano N, Okada T, Kayama K, et al. Delta-6 desaturase activity during the first year of life in preterm infants. Prostaglandins Leukot Essent Fatty Acids. 2016;115:8–11.

19 Najm S, Lofqvist C, Hellgren G, et al. Effects of a lipid emulsion containing fish oil on polyunsaturated fatty acid profiles, growth and morbidities in extremely premature infants: a randomized controlled trial. Clin Nutr ESPEN. 2017;20:17–23.

20 Collins CT, Makrides M, McPhee AJ, et al. Docosahexaenoic acid and bronchopulmonary dysplasia in preterm infants. N Engl J Med. 2017;376(13):1245–55.

21 Hellstrom A, Nilsson AK, Wackernagel D, et al. Effect of enteral lipid supplement on severe retinopathy of prematurity: a randomized clinical trial. JAMA Pediatr. 2021;175(4):359–67.

22 Wendel K, Pfeiffer HCV, Fugelseth DM, et al. Effects of nutrition therapy on growth, inflammation and metabolism in immature infants: a study protocol of a double-blind randomized controlled trial (ImNuT). BMC Pediatr. 2021;21(1):19.

23 Mihatsch W, Shamir R, van Goudoever JB, et al. ESPGHAN/ESPEN/ESPR/CSPEN guidelines on pediatric parenteral nutrition: guideline development process for the updated guidelines. Clin Nutr. 2018;37(6 Pt B):2306–8.

24 Agostoni C, Buonocore G, Carnielli VP, et al. Enteral nutrient supply for preterm infants: commentary from the European Society of Paediatric Gastroenterology, Hepatology and Nutrition Committee on Nutrition. J Pediatr Gastroenterol Nutr. 2010;50(1):85–91.

25 Wackernagel D, Bruckner A, Ahlsson F. Computer-aided nutrition – effects on nutrition and growth in preterm infants <32 weeks of gestation. Clin Nutr ESPEN. 2015;10(6):e234-e41.

Magnus Domellöf
Department of Clinical Sciences, Pediatrics
Umeå University
SE -901 85 Umeå
Sweden
magnus.domellof@umu.se

Published online: May 10, 2022

Embleton ND, Haschke F, Bode L (eds): Strategies in Neonatal Care to Promote Optimized Growth and Development: Focus on Low Birth Weight Infants. 96th Nestlé Nutrition Institute Workshop, May 2021. Nestlé Nutr Inst Workshop Ser. Basel, Karger, 2022, vol 96, pp 138–140 (DOI: 10.1159/000519404)

Summary on Personalized Nutrition of Preterm Infants

Mother's own milk should be the first choice when enteral nutrition starts, and banked human milk (HM) can be offered whenever mothers' own milk is not available. HM has a strong trophic effect on the immature gut, provides protection against necrotizing enterocolitis and late-onset sepsis, and might have beneficial effects on brain development. Banked HM has limitations like low protein content and unpredictable composition of other macro- and micronutrients. Neonatal caregivers should be aware of unpredictable composition of banked HM. For safe HM bank operation, international guidelines with regard to safety and nutrient screening have been published.

HM should be fortified with protein, energy, and micronutrients which are provided by commercially available multinutrient HM fortifiers. Due to the fear of contamination of powdered products with *Cronobacter sakazakii*, liquid fortifiers are widely used in the United States. They have the advantage to be completely sterile, and another benefit is easier mixing. The main downside of liquid fortifiers is their volume replacement of HM (about 16.7%). The recommendations on the amounts of enteral protein needed by preterm infants (3.5–4.5 g/kg/day) are based on the reference fetus and clinical trials which have recently been reviewed and form the basis of evidence-based guidelines. The presently available powdered and liquid HMFs add 1.4–1.8 g protein to 100 mL of HM. The protein:energy ratio in fortified HM is important because low energy supply results in increased oxidation of amino acids, which then serve as energy source. All cow's milk-based fortifiers try to copy the amino acid profile of HM; thus, the fortifiers' protein is spiked with amino acids. However, recently published evidence-based nutrition practice guidelines for preterm infants conclude that no recommendations can be made on protein quality (amino acid profile) in HMF because there are no studies in the literature. Metabolic balance studies and the stable isotope technology have been employed to estimate amino acid requirements of preterm infants. Recently calculated amino acid requirements which are based on amino acid gains of the fetus can serve as reference for advisable intakes/kg/day of preterm infants: requirements of extremely low birth weight (<500–1,000 g) and very low birth weight infants (1,000–15,000 g), are 77 and 30% higher than those of low birth weight infants growing from 1,900 to 2,400 g. The very high amino acid requirements of extremely low birth weight infants are a challenge for enteral nutrition. Amino acid profiles of present HMFs for preterm infants which are close to HM should be reconsidered: spiking HM fortifier protein with the amino acids which are presently undersupplied or providing targeted amino acid-based HM fortifiers is an option to further improve the amino acid profile in fortifiers.

In newer HM fortifiers, the amount of carbohydrates is reduced and replaced by lipids including small amounts of the omega-3 and omega-6 long-chain polyunsaturated fatty acids. Infants born very preterm miss out on the in utero transfer of those fatty acids that occurs during the third trimester. A number of studies have explored the impact of increasing the enteral intakes of omega-3 +/− omega-6 long chain polyunsaturated fatty acids to match fetal accretion rates in such infants. They have shown early transient improvements in vision and development, but with the use of omega-3 supplementation alone appearing to increase the incidence of bronchopulmonary dysplasia. A recent study of omega-3 + omega-6 supplementation demonstrated a significant reduction in the incidence of severe retinopathy of prematurity in a high-risk population, without apparent adverse effects.

As far as micronutrients are concerned, iron supplementation of low birth weight infants reduces the risk of behavioral problems. However, due to the risk of adverse effects, iron supplementation of very preterm infants in the NICU should be individualized, considering birth weight, postnatal age, diet, and serum ferritin concentrations. Sodium intakes should be minimized during the first 3 days of life in very preterm infants to avoid hypernatremia. However, after 4 days of age, sodium supplements can reduce hyponatremia and improve growth. Adequate enteral calcium, phosphorus, and vitamin D intakes are crucial for the prevention of osteopenia of prematurity. Screening of serum phosphate concentrations is useful.

Providing a HM fortifier once the preterm infant has started to suckle at the breast can be challenging for the mother and might shorten duration of the breastfeeding period. After hospital discharge, some mothers may not want to pump, fortify, and bottle-feed the fortifier-milk mixture any longer. The use of a finger feeder to administer a fortifier to preterm infants is a new method that enables mothers to exclusively breastfeed their infants and meet their nutritional needs. More than 67% of the infants accepted the device, and fortifier application during nursing went very well. Future efforts to enable fortification during breastfeeding must be linked to the development of ready-to-use devices, which contain liquid HM fortification portions. Early-life stress and even minor nutritional insufficiencies lastingly alter brain, behavior, and mental health, but still little is known about the exact working and interplay of these pathways. Over the last years, there has been increased attention to the prevention of the detrimental consequences of stressful experiences in early life. Stress reduction programs for both parents and their preterm children have been developed, and the advantages of family integrated care are being acknowledged increasingly. Although all nutrients are necessary for brain growth, key nutrients that support neurodevelopment include macronutrients such as fatty acids and proteins, and micronutrients such as iron, choline, folate, iodine, and vitamins. Nutritional supplementation studies in preterm infants have shown beneficial effects on neurocognitive development, even after adjusting for confounding factors (i.e., gestational age at delivery, birth weight, and comorbidities). Increased cumulative intakes of energy, protein, and lipids have been associated with better developmental outcomes.

Ferdinand Haschke

Published online: May 10, 2022

Embleton ND, Haschke F, Bode L (eds): Strategies in Neonatal Care to Promote Optimized Growth and Development: Focus on Low Birth Weight Infants. 96th Nestlé Nutrition Institute Workshop, May 2021. Nestlé Nutr Inst Workshop Ser. Basel, Karger, 2022, vol 96, pp 141–148 (DOI: 10.1159/000519396)

Importance of the Gut Microbiome in Preterm Infants

Christopher J. Stewart

Translational and Clinical Research Institute, Newcastle University, Newcastle upon Tyne, UK

Abstract

Birth represents the start of an incredible journey for the individual and the microbes which reside within and upon them. This interaction between human and microbe is essential for healthy development. Term infants are colonized by bacteria at birth, and thereafter the diet is the most important factor shaping the gut microbiome, in particular receipt of human milk. Human milk contains viable bacteria and numerous components that modulate the bacterial community, including human milk oligosaccharides (HMOs) which promote the growth of *Bifidobacterium* species. Notably, *Bifidobacterium* spp. are the primary bacterium used in probiotic supplements, owing to their association with positive outcomes in cohort studies and range of beneficial properties in mechanistic experiments. Preterm infants born <32 weeks' gestation encounter an unnatural beginning to life, with housing in "sterile" incubators, higher rates of caesarean delivery and antibiotic use, and complex nutritional provision. This reduces *Bifidobacterium* abundance and overall microbial diversity. However, this also presents an opportunity to use probiotics and prebiotics (e.g., HMOs) to restore "normal" development. Much work has focused in this area over the past two decades and, while more work is needed, there is promise in symbiotic intervention to modulate the microbiome and reduce disease in preterm infants.

Development of the Gut Microbiome in Term and Preterm Infants

Following birth, neonates are rapidly colonized by microbes that play fundamental roles in health and disease. To a bacterial cell, the human body is like a universe, with different planets (i.e., body sites) containing distinct atmospheres (i.e., temperature, oxygen levels, acidity, humidity, etc.) and resources (i.e., food sources and metals). This predisposes the body to colonization by specific microorganisms that are able to survive in that environment and use the available resources to replicate. The gut contains the largest density of microorganisms, termed the gut microbiome, which have important roles in protection from pathogens, immune system training, the breakdown of dietary compounds, and many other functions [1]. Over the first year of life, the infant gut microbiome is highly dynamic, providing a window of opportunity in which to seed a potentially beneficial microbiome and reduce the risk of early- and later-life diseases. In term infants, birth mode and breastfeeding are the most important variables for shaping the early life microbiome [2]. Infants born vaginally have a higher prevalence and relative abundance of *Bacteroides* spp., which an enteric bacterium and is most likely transferred via the fecal-oral route during delivery [3]. Receipt of human milk is the primary factor shaping the infant gut microbiome over the first year of life, increasing the relative abundance of *Bifidobacterium* spp. and reducing the relative abundance of pathobionts [2, 4]. Other factors reported to influence infant gut microbiome development include geographical location and having furry pets in the household [2]. However, such influences are only observed up to ~1.5 years of life, after which the gut microbiome becomes increasingly individualized and stable. This early life host-microbiome cross talk and immune development is hypothesized to have important roles in long-term health and is directly correlated to an increased risk of obesity, allergy, asthma, and other disorders later in life [5].

Preterm infants born <32 weeks of gestation encounter an unnatural beginning to life, with housing in "sterile" incubators, higher rates of caesarean delivery and antibiotic use, inability to feed at the breast, complex nutritional supplementation, and parenteral nutrition that bypasses the gastrointestinal tract. Such factors are necessary to maximize survival in this vulnerable population, but as a consequence, the gut microbiome and microbial-host cross talk is abnormal when compared to term infants [6]. In comparison to term infants, preterm infants have lower microbiome diversity and enrichment of pathobionts including *Staphylococcus*, *Klebsiella*, *Escherichia*, *Enterobacter*, and *Enterococcus*, and a reduction in potentially beneficial bacteria including *Lactobacillus* and *Bifidobacterium* [7].

Microbially Mediated Disease in Preterm Infants

Owing to an altered microbiome, coupled with an immature intestinal architecture (e.g., leaky gut) and an underdeveloped immune system, preterm infants are predisposed to intestinal diseases such as necrotizing enterocolitis (NEC). NEC is the leading cause of death in preterm infants surviving the initial days of life, where exaggerated inflammation cascades to epithelial damage, ischemia, and ultimately necrosis of the bowel. Around 50% of cases will require surgery and of those going to theatre, the survival rate is around 50%. It is likely there are numerous pathways underlying NEC pathogenesis that ultimately manifest in a common endpoint of intestinal necrosis. To this end, work is currently ongoing to characterize and better understand different NEC subtypes. Currently, the most well-characterized is the toll-like receptor (TLR)-4 pathway. Work by Hackam and Sodhi [8], as well as others, have shown that TLR4 expressed specifically on the surface of intestinal epithelial cells (and not immune cells), is activated when the gut is exposed to lipopolysaccharides (LPS) found on the outer membrane of Gram-negative bacteria. TLR4 is crucial for normal fetal development and, as such, is expressed in high levels during this period. Since LPS would not be expected in the gut during this period, activation of TLR4 receptors is not a problem; however, TLR4 expression remains high following premature birth. Once activated, it results in a three-pronged destructive process whereby (1) the nuclear factor kappa B (NF-κB) pathway is activated, leading to increased inflammation, (2) enterocyte destruction, and (3) failure to restore epithelial damage owning to reduced replication and migration of crypt-derived stem cells. This leads to increased translation of enteric bacteria and reduced blood flow to the site of damage, reflecting the common inflamed and necrotic pathology.

Late-onset sepsis (LOS) is another common disease of preterm infants, with greater prevalence but lower overall mortality when compared to NEC. While LOS is not solely a disease of intestinal origin, there is mounting evidence to support the gut as a common route for translocating bacteria. For example, common enteric bacteria of preterm infants, such as *Klebsiella* and *Escherichia*, are regularly identified as the causative agent in LOS [9]. There are also reports in preterm infants receiving dietary probiotics where the probiotic strain is detected in diagnostic blood culture [10]. Ward et al. [11] further showed the uropathogenic *Escherichia coli* strains detected in the infant gut could also be isolated in diagnostic blood culture.

Human Milk and Probiotics to Increase *Bifidobacterium* in Preterm Infants

Once a baby is born prematurely, maternal breast milk is the single most protective factor against NEC [12]. However, infants receiving mother's own milk still develop the disease, suggesting numerous other factors to be involved, including the variable composition of nutrients and other components of human milk. In addition, extremely preterm infants cannot be directly breastfed, necessitating expression, freezing, and nasogastric feeding. Human milk contains viable maternal bacteria that colonize the infant gut [13, 14], but expressed human milk delivered by nasogastric tube is enriched with potential pathogens and reduced levels of beneficial *Bifidobacterium* [15]. Human milk also contains an abundance of human milk oligosaccharides (HMOs), which are a family of structurally diverse sugars, absent from standard preterm formula milk [16]. HMOs are unbound and cannot be digested by the infant, so they reach the lower gastrointestinal tract intact where they act as growth substrates for specific bacteria, most notably *Bifidobacterium* [4]. While their primary role is likely to serve as a prebiotic, there is mounting evidence that they play important roles in epithelial function and immune development. Seminal work by Bode and colleagues [17] has shown a specific HMO, disialyllacto-*N*-tetraose (DSLNT), was associated with protection against NEC in humans, which was validated in a rat model [18]. This was recently supported by a large observational study of 33 NEC cases, where DSLNT could predict the risk of NEC with a sensitivity and specificity of 0.9 [19]. Separate work has shown that the HMO 2′-fucosyllactose (2′FL) reduced stimulation of TLR4, suppressing activation of the NF-κB inflammatory pathway and ameliorating LPS-stimulated inflammation [20]. While 2′-FL is the most abundant HMO in human milk, nonsecretor mothers lacking a functional FUT2 allele, who represent ~20% of the population, will lack or produce only trace levels of α1–2 fucosylated oligosaccharides. Notably, no association between 2′FL and NEC risk has been observed in cohort studies, and there is no report of maternal secretor status (i.e., 2′FL presence/absence in milk) as a factor that impacts the likelihood of developing NEC.

Given the importance of the gut microbiome in NEC and the improvements in sequencing technologies that allow bacteria to be surveyed, a large number of studies over the past decade have sequenced stool in preterm infants with NEC and matched controls. Despite improved understanding of preterm infant gut microbiome development, there has been no consistent bacterium or combination of bacteria that reproducibly associate with NEC onset. The most consistent associations are evident at the phylum level, with a higher abundance of proteobacteria found in infants who are diagnosed with NEC. On the other hand, there has been evidence that a higher bacterial diversity and higher *Bifidobacterium* spp. is associated with protection against NEC [9, 19, 21–25]. Recent work utilizing HMO profiling of mothers' milk and metagenomic sequencing of preterm infant gut microbiome showed the HMO composition in human milk was associated with altered microbiome development. Specifically, infants receiving low concentrations of DLSNT had reduced transition into mature microbiome community types which were dominant in *Bifidobacterium* spp. [20]. Such studies highlight the importance of diet-microbe-host interaction, but in observational studies utilizing clinical samples it is difficult to determine cause or effect. Possible models for further investigating this interaction at the preterm epithelial surface are proposed in a subsequent section. Animal models have also been used to investigate potential mechanisms, showing bacteria such as *Bifidobacterium* spp. may increase gut and immune maturation, which could reduce the risk of NEC in preterm infants [22].

The findings of enriched *Bifidobacterium* in healthy infants have led, in part, to an increased attention and use of probiotics within neonatal intensive care units. Despite this, human preterm probiotic trials have yielded inconsistent results, potentially reflecting the lack of knowledge to underpin probiotic choice, the optimal dosage, the timing and frequency to supplement, what other prebiotics are needed for probiotic colonization/replication and beneficial functioning, variable colonization rates, and cross-contamination between randomized groups [26]. Nonetheless, recent meta-analyses show that, overall, probiotics significantly reduce NEC, and their use is supported by the European Society for Paediatric Gastroenterology Hepatology and Nutrition Working Group for Probiotics and Prebiotics [27]. However, a recent clinical report from the American Academy of Pediatrics concluded that based on the current evidence and the lack of FDA regulation, they do not support the routine use of probiotics in preterm infants [28]. Such conflicting recommendations highlight the need for further work to optimize the use of probiotics in preterm infants.

Next-Generation Organoid Models for Studying Preterm Intestinal Health and Disease

Better understanding of the interaction between bacteria and infant gut epithelial cells holds incredibly exciting possibilities to better predict, diagnose, and manipulate the microbiome of preterm infants at risk of disease. Animal models have provided important advances; however, the microbiome varies significantly between different animal species, and thus the direct relevance and translation of findings into humans is challenging [29]. The anatomical differences between animal models and neonatal gut, as well as the inability to model extreme gut prematurity (i.e., <32 weeks of gestation), represent further limitations of animal models. To overcome these longstanding hurdles and advance upon associations by investigating underlying mechanisms, several groups have turned to human intestinal-derived organoids (HIOs). HIOs are generated from resected intestinal tissue by stimulating Lgr5+ stem cells isolated from intestinal crypts, and a recent method described a method for establishing lines from preterm infants [30]. HIOs remain morphologically representative of the segments of intestine they were taken from (e.g., ileum will be distinct from colon); are composed of all the major cell types of the intestinal epithelium (i.e., enterocyte, Paneth, goblet, neuroendocrine, and stem); and are physiologically active (i.e., secrete mucus and swell in response to enterotoxins) [29]. Furthermore, they retain the genetic and epigenetic susceptibility and immune programming of the host [31].

Owing to the different oxygen demands of host and microbe, until recently it was not possible to simultaneously co-culture viable HIOs with viable anaerobic enteric bacteria. However, several systems have recently been engineered to recapitulate the steep oxygen gradient across the epithelium. In such systems, the lumen (i.e., apical surface) is anaerobic to support the growth of bacteria, whereas the mucosa (i.e., basolateral surface) is oxygenated to maintain HIO viability. A microfluidic anaerobic intestine-on-a-chip has been developed and shown to sustain cell viability of anaerobic bacteria [32]. A different model called the organoid-anaerobe co-culture system can be setup using nonspecialist, commercially available equipment, and additionally allows easy adjustment of the basolateral oxygen concentration [33]. HIO co-culture systems may therefore be a robust and relevant model to systematically explore host responses to bacteria and other stimuli (e.g., milk bioactive components) in the human preterm intestine, allowing comprehensive mechanistic investigation of diet-host-microbiome interaction.

Concluding Remarks

Over the past decade, our understanding of the preterm infant gut microbiome has advanced immensely, but there is still much to learn. One challenge relating to clinical cohorts is the need for multi-site, multi-geographical cohorts, improving the power of observations and the generalizability of findings. Another challenge facing researchers relates to moving beyond the huge number of associations that have resulted from omic profiling of maternal and infant clinical samples, to understand cause or effect, and unravelling the potential mechanisms underpinning these associations. As demonstrated by the consistent observation of a single HMO, DLSNT, being higher in control infants across different studies (and thus cohorts), there is enormous potential for the development of novel biomarkers and therapeutic/preventative strategies. For instance, prioritizing donor milk high in DLSNT for preterm infants and/or supplementing the diet with synthesized DSLNT where required. Such possibilities, as well as other emerging therapies, require deeper understanding and optimization for use in preterm infants before being rolled out. The risk in considering only a single component of a complex system of diet-microbe-host interaction is epitomized with probiotics, where simply providing so-called beneficial bacteria without other components (e.g., prebiotics) to support their growth and beneficial functioning has failed to yield consistent and widespread improvements to outcomes for preterm infants. Nevertheless, personalized or stratified approaches to modulate the gut microbiome though symbiotics is one emerging area that holds genuine potential to reduce the risk of devastating disease in preterm infants.

Conflict of Interest Statement

C.J.S. declares performing consultancy for Astarte Medical and receiving lecture honoraria from Danone Early Life Nutrition and Nestlé Nutrition Institute but has no share options or other conflicts.

References

1   Young VB. The role of the microbiome in human health and disease: an introduction for clinicians. BMJ. 2017;356:j831.
2   Stewart CJ, Ajami NJ, O'Brien JL, et al. Temporal development of the gut microbiome in early childhood from the TEDDY study. Nature. 2018;562:583–8.
3   Korpela K, Helve O, Kolho KL, et al. Maternal fecal microbiota transplantation in cesarean-born infants rapidly restores normal gut microbial development: a proof-of-concept study. Cell. 2020;183:324–34.e5.
4   Vatanen T, Franzosa EA, Schwager R, et al. The human gut microbiome in early-onset type 1 diabetes from the TEDDY study. Nature. 2018;562:589–94.
5   Davis MK. Breastfeeding and Chronic Disease in Childhood and Adolescence. Pediatr Clin North Am. 2001;48:125–41.
6   Stewart C, Skeath T, Nelson A, et al. Preterm gut microbiota and metabolome following discharge from intensive care. Sci Rep. 2015;5:17141.
7   Masi AC, Stewart CJ. The role of the preterm intestinal microbiome in sepsis and necrotising enterocolitis. Early Hum Dev. 2019 Nov;138:104854.
8   Hackam DJ, Sodhi CP. Toll-like receptor – mediated intestinal inflammatory imbalance in the pathogenesis of necrotizing enterocolitis. Cell Mol Gastroenterol Hepatol. 2018;6:229–38.e1.
9   Stewart CJ, Embleton ND, Marrs ECL, et al. Longitudinal development of the gut microbiome and metabolome in preterm neonates with late onset sepsis and healthy controls. Microbiome. 2017;5:75.
10 Esaiassen E, Cavanagh P, Hjerde E, et al. *Bifidobacterium longum* subspecies *infantis* bacteremia in 3 extremely preterm infants receiving probiotics. Emerg Infect Dis. 2016;22:1664–6.
11 Ward DV, Scholz M, Zolfo M, et al. Metagenomic sequencing with strain-level resolution implicates uropathogenic *E. coli* in necrotizing enterocolitis and mortality in preterm infants. Cell Rep. 2016;14:2912–24.

12 Patel AL, Kim JH. Human milk and necrotizing enterocolitis. Semin Pediatr Surg. 2018;27:34–8.

13 Lackey KA, Williams JE, Meehan CL, et al. What's normal? Microbiomes in human milk and infant feces are related to each other but vary geographically: The INSPIRE Study. Front Nutr. 2019;6:45.

14 Stewart CJ, Marrs ECL, Nelson A, et al. Development of the preterm gut microbiome in twins at risk of necrotising enterocolitis and sepsis. PLoS One. 2013;8:e73465.

15 Moossavi S, Sepehri S, Robertson B, et al. Composition and variation of the human milk microbiota are influenced by maternal and early-life factors. Cell Host Microbe. 2019;25:324–35.e4.

16 Bode L. Human milk oligosaccharides: every baby needs a sugar mama. Glycobiology. 2012;22:1147–62.

17 Autran CA, Kellman BP, Kim JH, et al. Human milk oligosaccharide composition predicts risk of necrotising enterocolitis in preterm infants. Gut. 2018;67:1064–70.

18 Jantscher-Krenn E, Zherebtsov M, Nissan C, et al. The human milk oligosaccharide disialyllacto-N-tetraose prevents necrotising enterocolitis in neonatal rats. Gut. 2012;61:1417–25.

19 Masi A, Embleton N, Lamb C, et al. Human milk oligosaccharide DSLNT and gut microbiome in preterm infants predicts necrotising enterocolitis. Gut. 2020 Dec 16;gutjnl-2020-322771. doi: 10.1136/gutjnl-2020-322771.

20 He Y, Liu S, Kling DE, et al. The human milk oligosaccharide 2′-fucosyllactose modulates CD14 expression in human enterocytes, thereby attenuating LPS-induced inflammation. Gut. 2016;65:33–46.

21 Stewart CJ, Embleton ND, Marrs ECL, et al. Temporal bacterial and metabolic development of the preterm gut reveals specific signatures in health and disease. Microbiome. 2016;4:67.

22 Fanning S, Hall LJ, Cronin M, et al. Bifidobacterial surface-exopolysaccharide facilitates commensal-host interaction through immune modulation and pathogen protection. Proc Natl Acad Sci USA. 2012;109:2108–13.

23 Olm MR, Bhattacharya N, Crits-Christoph A, et al. Necrotizing enterocolitis is preceded by increased gut bacterial replication, *Klebsiella*, and fimbriae-encoding bacteria. Sci Adv. 2019;5:5727–38.

24 Pammi M, Cope J, Tarr PI, et al. Intestinal dysbiosis in preterm infants preceding necrotizing enterocolitis: a systematic review and meta-analysis. Microbiome. 2017;5:31.

25 Stewart CJ, Fatemizadeh R, Parsons P, et al. Using formalin fixed paraffin embedded tissue to characterize the preterm gut microbiota in necrotising enterocolitis and spontaneous isolated perforation using marginal and diseased tissue. BMC Microbiol. 2019;19:52.

26 Patel RM, Underwood MA. Probiotics and necrotizing enterocolitis. Semin Pediatr Surg. 2018;27:39–46.

27 van den Akker CHP, van Goudoever JB, Shamir R, et al. Probiotics and preterm infants: a position paper by the European Society for Paediatric Gastroenterology Hepatology and Nutrition Committee on Nutrition and the European Society for Paediatric Gastroenterology Hepatology and Nutrition Working Group for Probiotics and Prebiotics. J Pediatr Gastroenterol Nutr. 2020;70:664–80.

28 Poindexter B. Use of probiotics in preterm infants. Pediatrics. 2021;147:e2021051485.

29 Blutt SE, Crawford SE, Ramani S, et al. Engineered Human Gastrointestinal Cultures to Study the Microbiome and Infectious Diseases. Cell Mol Gastroenterol Hepatol. 2017;5:241–51.

30 Stewart CJ, Estes MK, Ramani S. Establishing human intestinal enteroid/organoid lines from preterm infant and adult tissue. Methods Mol Biol. 2121;185–198.

31 Kraiczy J, Nayak KM, Howell KJ, et al. DNA methylation defines regional identity of human intestinal epithelial organoids and undergoes dynamic changes during development. Gut. 2019;68:49–61.

32 Jalili-Firoozinezhad S, Gazzaniga FS, Calamari EL, et al. Complex human gut microbiome cultured in anaerobic human intestine chips. bioRxiv. 2018;421404. doi:10.1101/421404

33 Fofanova TY, Stewart C, Auchtung JM, et al. A novel human enteroid-anaerobe co-culture system to study microbial-host interaction under physiological hypoxia. bioRxiv. 2019;555755. doi: 10.1101/555755.

Christopher J. Stewart
Translational and Clinical Research Institute
Faculty of Medical Sciences
Newcastle University
3rd Floor Leech Building
Newcastle NE2 4HH
UK
Christopher.Stewart@newcastle.ac.uk

Published online: May 10, 2022

Embleton ND, Haschke F, Bode L (eds): Strategies in Neonatal Care to Promote Optimized Growth and Development: Focus on Low Birth Weight Infants. 96th Nestlé Nutrition Institute Workshop, May 2021. Nestlé Nutr Inst Workshop Ser. Basel, Karger, 2022, vol 96, pp 149–159 (DOI: 10.1159/000519388)

Selected Human Milk Oligosaccharides Added to Infant Formulas for Term Infants

Hania Szajewska

Department of Paediatrics, Medical University of Warsaw, Warsaw, Poland

Abstract

The benefits of breastfeeding, such as reduced risk of gastrointestinal and respiratory tract infections, depend largely on the presence of bioactive compounds in breast milk, including human milk oligosaccharides (HMOs). The presence of HMOs represents one of the largest differences in composition between breast milk and infant formula. Currently, progress in biotechnology allows the production of selected HMOs such as 2′-fucosyllactose (2′-FL) and lacto-N-neotetraose (LNnT), which are increasingly being added to infant formulas to narrow the difference between breast milk and formula. It is important to differentiate HMOs naturally occurring in human breast milk from those biotechnologically produced, which, while identical to HMOs in breast milk, do not originate from breast milk. This chapter summarizes basic facts about HMOs, findings from observational studies assessing the relationship between specific HMOs and clinical effects, and evidence from randomized controlled trials with structures identical to HMOs in breast milk added to infant formulas. Overall, the findings from some recently published trials provide reassurance that infant formulas supplemented with selected structures identical to HMOs, specifically 2′-FL with/out LNnT, are safe and well tolerated, and may have favorable effects on some health outcomes and medication usage. Further studies are needed. © 2022 S. Karger AG, Basel

Introduction

The benefits of breastfeeding, such as reduced risk of gastrointestinal and respiratory tract infections [1], depend largely on the presence of bioactive compounds in breast milk, including human milk oligosaccharides (HMOs) [2]. Over the past few years, HMOs have become one of the hot topics of research in infant nutrition. It results from the development of analytical methods that allow better understanding of the structures and properties of HMOs. Furthermore, at least some HMOs can be produced in large quantities using modern biotechnological methods. Some of these are added to infant formulas to narrow the gap between breast milk and infant formula. This article summarizes basic facts on HMOs and findings from (1) observational studies assessing the relationship between specific HMOs and clinical effects, and (2) randomized controlled trials (RCTs) with selected HMOs added to infant formulas. For the latter, a search of PubMed and Cochrane library was performed from 2015 to April 2021.

Human Milk Oligosaccharides

A detailed discussion of HMOs is beyond the scope of this article but can be found elsewhere [3, 4]. In brief, HMOs are complex carbohydrates that include five monosaccharides: glucose, galactose, N-acetylglucosamine, fucose, and sialic acid. In terms of quantity, HMOs are the third largest solid component of breast milk (only lactose and fats are present in greater amounts). It is estimated that breast milk contains about 150–200 structurally distinct HMOs, although the exact number is unknown. Each mother produces a specific HMO set, which is genetically determined (similar to blood groups). HMOs have no nutritional value for the infant. They primarily act as prebiotics by promoting healthy gut microbiota composition and serving as a selective source of nutrition for some microorganisms, mainly *Bifidobacterium infantis*, *Bifidobacterium bifidum*, and *Bifidobacterium breve*, inhabiting the gastrointestinal tract. These microorganisms "repay" the host by modifying the microbiota and contributing to a reduction in the risk of diseases, especially gastrointestinal infections. Additionally, HMOs act as antimicrobial agents by preventing pathogen adhesion to epithelial cells. HMOs are also involved in immune function acting as intestinal epithelial cell modulators, by enhancing maturation of the intestinal mucosa and intestinal epithelial barrier function, and as immunomodulators directly or indirectly modulating the immune system.

Findings from Observational Studies on Specific HMOs and Clinical Effects

In addition to a number of in vitro studies documenting the effects of HMOs such as immunomodulatory activity against viruses (influenza, rotavirus, respiratory syncytial virus, norovirus) [5], observational human studies suggest an association between the levels of both total HMOs and specific HMOs in breast milk and clinical effects in infants. Among others, the studies analyzed the associations between HMOs and outcomes such as [3]:

- Gastrointestinal infections – a lower risk of *Campylobacter jejuni*-induced diarrhea in children who received breast milk containing large amounts of 2′-fucosyllactose (2′-FL) and a lower risk of *Calicivirus*-induced diarrhea in children receiving milk with a high content of another fucosylated HMO, lacto-*N*-difucohexaose I, was shown [6]
- Allergies – the results of studies are not conclusive [7–9]; however, preliminary data suggest a link between fucosylated HMOs (2′-FL) and a reduction in the risk of allergies, especially in infants born via caesarean section [10]
- Necrotizing enterocolitis – a link between low levels of disialyl-lacto-*N*-tetraose in breast milk and the risk of necrotizing enterocolitis in premature infants was documented [11, 12]
- Sepsis – high concentrations of fucosyl-disialyllacto-*N*-hexaose in breast milk were associated with a reduced risk of death in very low birth weight infants with sepsis [13]
- Overweight/obesity – the results of a small study showed differences in the HMO composition of breast milk from mothers of breastfed infants with normal and excessive weight gain; in the latter case, a higher 2′-FL content was found [14, 15]

Association, however, is not causation. Observational studies are not sufficient for proving that any specific HMOs would alter health. Still, the findings are important, as they indicate directions for further research.

Structures Identical to HMOs Added to Infant Formulas

Until recently, obtaining HMOs was very difficult. However, biotechnological methods, including microbial fermentation using genetically engineered microorganisms *E. coli* and yeast [16], allow the manufacture of selected HMOs, including 2′-FL and lacto-*N*-neotetraose (LNnT), in very large quantities [17]. Since 2016, 2′-FL and LNnT have also been added to some infant formulas. Two leading institutions providing opinions on food-related issues (European Food Safety Authority [EFSA] [18] and Food and Drug Administration [FDA]) [19],

Table 1. Examples of commercially available structures identical to HMO in breast milk

2'-fucosyllactose	2'-FL
Lacto-N-neotetraose	LNnT
Lacto-N-tetraose	LNT
3-fucosyllactose	3-FL
Difucosyllactose	DiFL (or DFL or LDFT)
Lacto-N-triose II	LNT-II
Lacto-N-fucopentaose I	LNFP I
Lacto-N-fucopentaose III	LNFP III
Lacto-N-fucopentaose V	LNFP V
6'-sialyllactose	6'-SL
3'-sialyllactose	3'-SL

independently of each other, have confirmed the safety of 2'-FL and LNnT when added alone or in combination to infant, follow-on, and young child formula. Other HMOs are also available (Table 1) [20]. However, it is unlikely that all HMOs found in breast milk can be produced in the near future (or are even needed).

Terminology

It is important to differentiate HMOs naturally occurring in human breast milk from those biotechnologically produced, which, while identical to HMOs in breast milk, do not originate from breast milk. Those biotechnologically manufactured HMOs are sometimes called "*synthetic HMOs*" [21] or "*human-identical milk oligosaccharides*" [22] or "*artificial HMOs*" [23] or "*HMO analogues*" [24]. Another option is the term "structures identical to HMOs." However, there is no consensus regarding the terminology, and further discussions are needed to ensure general agreement and scientific clarity in communication.

Findings from RCTs of Infant Formulas Supplemented with 2'-FL and LNnT

Table 2 summarizes the key results of RCTs published as full papers (as of April 2021) assessing the safety and efficacy of infant formulas supplemented with 2'-FL with or without LNnT.

2'-FL Supplementation
A 2015 RCT by Marriage et al. [25] evaluated the effects of 2'-FL-supplemented infant formula on weight gain per day from day of life 14 to 119 (primary end-

Table 2. Infant formulas supplemented with 2'-FL with or without LNnT – summary of trials with clinical outcomes

Author	Design	Population	Interventions	Comparison	Primary endpoint	Key results
Puccio et al. [27]	RCT, DB	Healthy term born infants, recruitment ≤14 days of age	IF + 2'-FL 1 g/L + LNnT 0.5 g/L for 6 months (n = 88); observation – 12 months	IF (n = 87)	Growth indices	Age-appropriate growth (primary endpoint); good tolerance; reduced risk of some infections and reduced use of some drugs (antibiotics, antipyretics) – secondary endpoints, parent-reported, requiring confirmation
Marriage et al. [25]	RCT, DB	Healthy, term born infants, recruitment 0–5 days of age; birth weight ≥2,490 g	IF + GOS 2.2 g/L + 2'-FL 0.2 g/L (n = 62)	IF + GOS 2.4 g/L (n = 68); reference group – breastfed infants (n = 65)	Growth indices	Age-appropriate growth; good tolerance
Goehring et al. [26] – cohort from the study above			IF + GOS 1.4 g/L + 2'-FL 1 g/L (n = 59)			Selected immunological parameters in groups receiving IF with 2'-FL similar to those seen in exclusively breastfed infants
Storm et al. [32]	RCT, DB	2 weeks of age (±5 days)	100% whey pHF + 2'-FL + B. lactis (n = 30)	100% whey pHF + B. lactis (n = 33)	Tolerance (using the IGSQ)	Well tolerated as confirmed by IGSQ
Nowak-Węgrzyn et al. [33]	CT	Children with cow's milk protein allergy (2 mo – 4 y); n = 64.	100% whey-based EHF + 2'-FL+LNnT	100% whey- based EHF	Hypoallerge-nicity and safety	Hypoallergenicity of test formula confirmed

2'-FL, 2'-fucosyllactose; B. lactis, Bifidobacterium animalis ssp lactis strain Bb12; CT, clinical trial; EHT, extensively hydrolyzed formula; FOS, fructooligosaccharides; GOS, galactooligosaccharides; IGSQ, Infant Gastrointestinal Symptom Questionnaire; IF, infant formula; LNnT, lacto-N-neotetraose; pHF, partially hydrolyzed formula; RCT, randomized controlled trial.

point) as well as tolerance and other anthropometric measures (secondary outcomes). Healthy infants born of a single pregnancy, with a birth weight ≥2,490 g, were eligible for the study. Infants meeting the inclusion criteria were randomly assigned to one of 3 groups in which they received: (1) infant formula containing galactooligosaccharides, with an energy value of 64.3 kcal/100 mL; (2) the same formula containing additional 2'-FL in the amount of 0.2 g/L, or (3) the same formula containing additional 2'-FL in the amount of 1 g/L. The reference group consisted of infants who met the eligibility criteria but were exclusively breastfed. The intervention, exclusive feeding of formula or breast milk, lasted until 119 days of age. Baseline clinical and demographic characteristics did not differ significantly between the intervention groups. Similar increases in weight, body length, and head circumference were found in all study groups, with growth parameters in the formula-fed groups similar to those found in exclusively breastfed infants. 2'-FL-supplemented formula was well tolerated. At 42 days of life, relative absorption of 2'-FL in the experimental formula groups was similar to that seen in breastfed infants.

In another publication [26], some of the same authors presented the results of an evaluation of the profiles of proinflammatory cytokines (TNF-α, IL-1α, IL-1β, IL-6) and anti-inflammatory IL-1ra in circulating plasma from a subset of the subjects in the original RCT. In both groups receiving 2'-FL-supplemented formula, compared to the control formula group, the levels of cytokines tested were lower and similar to those observed in breastfed infants. In supernatants of human peripheral blood mononuclear cell cultures following ex vivo stimulation by RSV44 viruses, the 2'-FL-supplemented formula group did not differ significantly from the breastfed group. There was also no difference between the two groups in any of the cytokines tested. However, the levels of some cytokines were higher in the control formula group. The clinical significance of the observed differences remains to be clarified.

2'-FL and LNnT Supplementation

A 2017 RCT by Puccio et al. [27] assessed the impact of infant formula supplemented with 2'-FL and LNnT on growth, tolerance, and morbidity. Healthy infants born at term, recruited at the age of ≤14 days, were eligible for the study. Children meeting the inclusion criteria were randomly assigned to one of 2 groups in which they received intact-protein, cow's milk-based infant formula containing 2'-FL (1 g/L) and LNnT (0.5 g/L) (n = 88) or the same infant formula without supplementation (n = 87). The intervention lasted 6 months; then, all infants received standard follow-up formula without HMOs from 6 to 12 months. Baseline clinical and demographic characteristics did not differ significantly between the study groups. Both groups showed similar weight gain in the

4th month of life (primary endpoint) as well as similar other anthropometric parameters (body weight and length, head circumference, and BMI – all expressed as *z*-scores) measured throughout the observation period. Gastrointestinal tolerance was similar in both groups except for softer stool in the 2′-FL- and LNnT-supplemented formula group at 2 months. In addition, in the group fed with 2′-FL- and LNnT-supplemented formula, compared to the group fed with standard formula, there was a lower risk of parent-reported adverse events identified a priori and less medication use (secondary endpoints), including:

- Lower risk of bronchitis throughout all examined time intervals (assessed at 0–4, 0–6, and 0–12 months of life)
- Lower risk of lower respiratory tract infections (assessed at 0–12 months of life)
- Lower use of antipyretics (assessed at 0–4 months of life)
- Less use of antibiotics (assessed at 0–6 and 0–12 months of life)

The results regarding the lower risk of certain diseases and the lower use of medications require confirmation because they were parent-reported secondary endpoints (although verified by the study team). However, the impact of 2′-FL and LNnT supplementation on the use of antibiotics, which was reduced by 31% (relative risk 0.69, 95% CI 0.51–0.93), is important. Several studies have documented the links between early-life antibiotic therapy and the risk of disease (including obesity and allergies) in later life [28–30]. Antibiotic administration by itself is neither necessary nor sufficient as a cause of these diseases. However, its potential role cannot be ignored, and every intervention which reduces the use of antibiotics is worth considering.

Later, it was reported that reduced overall medication use (antipyretics and antibiotics) may be linked to the gut microbiota types. In particular, formula-fed infants who demonstrated fecal community type with Bifidobacteriaceae at high abundance at 3 months were less likely to require antibiotics during the first year than those with fecal community type with less abundant Bifidobacteriaceae [31].

Protein Hydrolysates Supplemented with 2′-FL and LNnT
At the time of the writing of this chapter, the results of 2 trials published as full papers were available, in which 2′-FL and LNnT were added to partially or extensively hydrolyzed formulas.

Whey-Based Partially Hydrolyzed Infant Formula with *Bifidobacterium lactis* and 2′-FL
In a 2019 RCT by Storm et al. [32], in which infants less than 2 weeks of age were eligible, the effect of using a whey-based (100%), partially hydrolyzed infant for-

mula supplemented with *Bifidobacterium animalis* ssp *lactis* strain Bb12 (control group; $n = 33$) was assessed for 6 weeks compared to the same hydrolysate containing additionally 2′-FL (experimental group; $n = 30$). A similar tolerance was found for both preparations assessed using the Infant Gastrointestinal Symptom Questionnaire (IGSQ). This questionnaire included bowel movements, vomiting, spitting, crying, and fussiness.

Whey-Based Extensively Hydrolyzed Infant Formula Containing 2′-FL and LNnT

A 2019 clinical trial by Nowak-Węgrzyn et al. [33] involving 67 children aged 2 months to 4 years with cow's milk protein allergy confirmed the hypoallergenicity of a whey-based (100%) extensively hydrolyzed infant (test) formula containing 2′-FL and LNnT. All children were assessed by double-blind, placebo-controlled food challenges to the test and control formulas, in random order. The product is considered to meet hypoallergenic conditions if it is well tolerated by at least 90% of patients (with a 95% confidence interval). The outcome of the DBPCFC in response to the test and control formulas confirmed the hypoallergenicity of the test formula.

Infants with cow's milk protein allergy may be at higher risk of infections. The findings of the CINNAMON study (ClinicalTrials.gov Identifier: NCT03085134; so far only presented in abstract form) demonstrated that children with cow's milk allergy fed a whey-based (100%) extensively hydrolyzed infant formula containing 2′-FL and LNnT with a reduced protein content (2.2 g/100 kcal) compared with those fed an un-supplemented formula with a higher protein content (2.5 g/100 kcal) had similar growth and tolerated well both formulas. Children fed 2′-FL- and LNnT-supplemented formula appeared to have a reduced risk of respiratory infections and reduced use of antibiotics and antipyretics; however, the differences between groups were not significant.

Further Trials Are Needed and Are Underway

At the time of the writing of this chapter, there were at least 13 interventional studies registered in ClinicalTrials.gov to evaluate various structures identical to HMOs in the pediatric population. These studies were at various stages (i.e., recruiting, completed). Among them, there is an RCT evaluating a mixture of five of the most commonly occurring HMOs in breast milk, i.e. 2′-FL, 2′,3-di-fucosyllactose, lacto-*N*-tetraose, 3′-sialyllactose, and 6′-sialyllactose. As no single ingredient is likely to act as a magic bullet, combining those with proven effects in one product brings infant formula closer to human breast milk and is justified. However, safety and clinical effects are still to be documented.

To ensure the quality of infant nutritional studies, standards for conducting such studies have been in development [34–36]. The most recent example is the document published in *JAMA Pediatrics* [35]. One of the questions asked was how to ensure the validity of clinical trials of breast milk substitutes while protecting trial participants, particularly with regard to breastfeeding. In line with the document, if the trial aims to demonstrate adequate infant growth and tolerance of a new breast milk substitute, participating infants should be fully breast milk-substitute-fed, and the decision not to use breast milk should be firmly established prior to enrollment in the trial. Both intention-to-treat and prespecified per protocol analyses are recommended. If the trial aims to generate data to support a nutrition or health claim, some infants will be receiving breast milk at enrollment, and it is important to demonstrate adequate support for breastfeeding. Only intention-to-treat analysis is recommended. While not addressed in the above document, one important issue when designing the study is to define what is an important difference between groups, i.e. minimal clinically important difference (MCID). This is defined as *"the smallest amount an outcome must change to be meaningful to patients"* [37]. Trivial differences between groups can become statistically significant but should be interpreted with caution in the context of MCID.

Conclusions

Research on HMOs is one of the hot topics in infant nutrition. Progress in biotechnology nowadays allows the production of at least some structures identical to HMOs to supplement infant formulas. Overall, the findings from some recently published trials, along with the EFSA and FDA opinions, provide reassurance that infant formulas supplemented with selected structures identical to HMOs, specifically 2′-FL with/out LNnT, are safe and well tolerated, and may have favorable effects on some health outcomes and medication usage. Further studies are needed. While awaiting new evidence, it seems reasonable to discuss with care providers current evidence regarding HMOs and structures identical to HMOs added to infant formulas and let them decide whether the expected benefits are in line with their expectations and worth the costs incurred. Evidence presented in this review should facilitate such discussion.

Conflict of Interest Statement

H.S. has participated as a consultant and/or speaker for companies manufacturing infant formulas, i.e. Danone, Else Nutrition, Hipp, Mead Johnson/RB Health, Nestlé, Nestlé Nutrition Institute.

References

1 Victora CG, Bahl R, Barros AJ, et al. Lancet Breastfeeding Series Group. Breastfeeding in the 21st century: epidemiology, mechanisms, and lifelong effect. Lancet. 2016;387:475–90.
2 Ballard O, Morrow AL. Human milk composition: nutrients and bioactive factors. Pediatr Clin North Am. 2013;60:49–74.
3 Triantis V, Bode L, van Neerven RJJ. Immunological effects of human milk oligosaccharides. Front Pediatr. 2018;6:190.
4 Walsh C, Lane JA, van Sinderen D, Hickey RM. Human milk oligosaccharides: shaping the infant gut microbiota and supporting health. J Funct Foods. 2020 Sep;72:104074.
5 Moore RE, Xu LL, Townsend SD. Prospecting human milk oligosaccharides as a defense against viral infections. ACS Infect Dis. 2021 Feb;12;7(2):254–63.
6 Morrow AL, Ruiz-Palacios GM, Altaye M, et al. Human milk oligosaccharides are associated with protection against diarrhea in breast-fed infants. J Pediatr. 2004 Sep;145(3):297–303.
7 Seppo AE, Autran CA, Bode L, Järvinen KM. Human milk oligosaccharides and development of cow's milk allergy in infants. J Allergy Clin Immunol. 2017 Feb;139(2):708–11.e5.
8 Miliku K, Robertson B, Sharma AK, et al. CHILD Study Investigators, Bode L, Azad MB. Human milk oligosaccharide profiles and food sensitization among infants in the CHILD Study. Allergy. 2018 Oct;73(10):2070–73.
9 Lodge CJ, Lowe AJ, Milanzi E, et al. Human milk oligosaccharide profiles and allergic disease up to 18 years. J Allergy Clin Immunol. 2021 Mar;147(3):1041–48.
10 Sprenger N, Odenwald H, Kukkonen AK, et al. FUT2-dependent breast milk oligosaccharides and allergy at 2 and 5 years of age in infants with high hereditary allergy risk. Eur J Nutr. 2017 Apr;56(3):1293–301.
11 Autran CA, Kellman BP, Kim JH, et al. Human milk oligosaccharide composition predicts risk of necrotising enterocolitis in preterm infants. Gut. 2018 Jun;67(6):1064–70.
12 Masi AC, Embleton ND, Lamb CA, et al. Human milk oligosaccharide DSLNT and gut microbiome in preterm infants predicts necrotising enterocolitis. Gut. 2020 Dec 16:gutjnl-2020–322771.

13 Torres Roldan VD, Urtecho SM, Gupta J, et al. Human milk oligosaccharides and their association with late-onset neonatal sepsis in Peruvian very-low-birth-weight infants. Am J Clin Nutr. 2020 Jul 1;112(1):106–12.
14 Larsson MW, Lind MV, Laursen RP, et al. Human milk oligosaccharide composition is associated with excessive weight gain during exclusive breastfeeding-an explorative study. Front Pediatr. 2019 Jul 18;7:297.
15 Lagström H, Rautava S, Ollila H, et al. Associations between human milk oligosaccharides and growth in infancy and early childhood. Am J Clin Nutr. 2020 Apr 1;111(4):769–78.
16 Salminen S, Stahl B, Vinderola G, Szajewska H. Infant formula supplemented with biotics: current knowledge and future perspectives. Nutrients. 2020 Jun 30;12(7):1952.
17 Walsh C, Lane JA, van Sinderen D, Hickey RM. From lab bench to formulated ingredient: characterization, production, and commercialization of human milk oligosaccharides. J Funct Foods. 2020;72:104052.
18 EFSA NDA Panel (EFSA Panel on Dietetic Products, Nutrition and Allergies), 2015. Scientific opinion on the safety of 2′-O-fucosyllactose as a novel food ingredient pursuant to Regulation (EC) No 258/97. EFSA J 2015;13(7):4184.
19 http://www.accessdata.fda.gov/scripts/ fdcc/?set=GRASNotices
20 Bych K, Mikš MH, Johanson T, et al. Production of HMOs using microbial hosts – from cell engineering to large scale production. Curr Opin Biotechnol. 2019 Apr;56:130–7.
21 Akkerman R, Faas MM, de Vos P. Non-digestible carbohydrates in infant formula as substitution for human milk oligosaccharide functions: effects on microbiota and gut maturation. Crit Rev Food Sci Nutr. 2019;59(9):1486–97.
22 Phipps KR, Baldwin N, Lynch B, et al. Safety evaluation of a mixture of the human-identical milk oligosaccharides 2′-fucosyllactose and difucosyllactose. Food Chem Toxicol. 2018 Oct;120:552–65.
23 Morozov V, Hansman G, Hanisch FG, et al. Human milk oligosaccharides as promising antivirals. Mol Nutr Food Res. 2018 Mar;62(6):e1700679.

24 Bering SB. Human milk oligosaccharides to prevent gut dysfunction and necrotizing enterocolitis in preterm neonates. Nutrients. 2018;10(10):1461.

25 Marriage BJ, Buck RH, Goehring KC, et al. Infants fed a lower calorie formula with 2'-FL show growth and 2'-FL uptake like breast-fed infants. J Pediatr Gastroenterol Nutr. 2015 Dec;61(6):649–58.

26 Goehring KC, Marriage BJ, Oliver JS, et al. Similar to those who are breastfed, infants fed a formula containing 2'-fucosyllactose have lower inflammatory cytokines in a randomized controlled trial. J Nutr. 2016 Dec;146(12):2559–66.

27 Puccio G, Alliet P, Cajozzo C, et al. Effects of infant formula with human milk oligosaccharides on growth and morbidity: a randomized multicenter trial. J Pediatr Gastroenterol Nutr. 2017 Apr;64(4):624–31.

28 Aversa Z, Atkinson EJ, Schafer MJ, et al. Association of infant antibiotic exposure with childhood health outcomes. Mayo Clin Proc. 2021 Jan;96(1):66–77.

29 Baron R, Taye M, der Vaart IB, et al. The relationship of prenatal antibiotic exposure and infant antibiotic administration with childhood allergies: a systematic review. BMC Pediatr. 2020 Jun;20(1):312.

30 Baron R, Taye M, Besseling-van der Vaart I, et al. SAWANTI working group. The relationship of prenatal and infant antibiotic exposure with childhood overweight and obesity: a systematic review. J Dev Orig Health Dis. 2019 Nov;18:1–15.

31 Berger B, Porta N, Foata F, et al. Linking human milk oligosaccharides, infant fecal community types, and later risk to require antibiotics. mBio. 2020 Mar;11(2):e03196–19.

32 Storm HM, Shepard J, Czerkies LM, et al. 2'-Fucosyllactose is well tolerated in a 100% whey, partially hydrolyzed infant formula with *Bifidobacterium lactis*: a randomized controlled trial. Glob Pediatr Health. 2019 Mar;6:2333794X19833995.

33 Nowak-Wegrzyn A, Czerkies L, Reyes K, et al. Confirmed hypoallergenicity of a novel whey-based extensively hydrolyzed infant formula containing two human milk oligosaccharides. Nutrients. 2019 Jun;11(7)pii:E1447.

34 Fewtrell MS. Clinical safety assessment of infant nutrition. Ann Nutr Metab. 2012;60(3):200–3.

35 Koletzko B, Fewtrell M, Gibson R, et al. Consensus Group on Outcome Measures Made in Paediatric Enteral Nutrition Clinical Trials (COMMENT); Early Nutrition Project. Core data necessary for reporting clinical trials on nutrition in infancy. Ann Nutr Metab. 2015;66(1):31–5.

36 Jarrold K, Helfer B, Eskander M, et al. Guidance for the conduct and reporting of clinical trials of breast milk substitutes. JAMA Pediatr. 2020 Sep;174(9):874–81.

37 McGlothlin AE, Lewis RJ. Minimal clinically important difference: defining what really matters to patients. JAMA. 2014 Oct;312(13):1342–3.

Hania Szajewska
Department of Paediatrics
Medical University of Warsaw
Żwirki i Wigury 63A
PL -02-091 Warsaw
Poland
hszajewska@wum.edu.pl

Published online: May 10, 2022

Embleton ND, Haschke F, Bode L (eds): Strategies in Neonatal Care to Promote Optimized Growth and Development: Focus on Low Birth Weight Infants. 96th Nestlé Nutrition Institute Workshop, May 2021. Nestlé Nutr Inst Workshop Ser. Basel, Karger, 2022, vol 96, pp 160–165 (DOI: 10.1159/000519390)

Microbiota and Human Milk Oligosaccharides in Premature Infants

Jean-Michel Hascoët[a]   Yipu Chen[b]

[a]Université de Lorraine and Maternité Régionale Universitaire A. Pinard, CHRU, Nancy, France; [b]Nestlé Product Technology Center – Nutrition, Vevey, Switzerland

Abstract

Gut microbiota plays an important role in infants' health. The prevalence of bifidobacteria in the gastrointestinal tract of term breastfed infants has been associated with reduced infection rates compared with formula-fed infants. However, few studies evaluated microbiota in premature infants. In an observational study of 577 preterm newborns born below 32 weeks gestation, gut microbiota was not driven by bifidobacteria but could be classified into six different clusters with regard to the most abundant bacteria present. Clusters were related to infants' maturity, perinatal determinants, and were associated with short- and long-term outcome. In another study, the effects of caesarean birth on infant gut microbiota could be alleviated by human milk oligosaccharides (HMOs) in mothers' milk. In addition, 58 infants fed with a formula enriched with 2 HMOs had microbiota closer to breastfed infants than 63 infants receiving the same formula without HMOs. The question then arose of the benefit of HMO supplementation for microbiota in premature infants. Thus, a multicenter randomized controlled intervention study of the effect of a liquid supplement containing 2 HMOs was set up. Ongoing data analysis will evaluate gastrointestinal tolerance parameters, intake of HMOs from human milk, long-term growth outcomes, fecal microbiota, and fecal biomarkers of gut maturation and immunity. © 2022 S. Karger AG, Basel

It is now well recognized that gut microbiota plays an important role in the health of infants. Breastfed term infants have a gut microbiota that is dominated by bifidobacteria, whereas formula-fed infants have a more heterogeneous composition, with comparatively lower levels of bifidobacteria [1, 2]. Diet composition significantly impacts the development of term born infants' gut microbiota [3]. The prevalence of bifidobacteria in the gastrointestinal tract of term breastfed infants has been associated with reduced infection rates and less allergy manifestation as compared with formula-fed infants [1, 4]. However, few data are available to support microbiota composition and its impact on premature and very premature infants' health. In the EPIFLORE study, a prospective observational cohort study that included stool sample collection within the fourth week after birth in 577 preterm newborns born below 32 weeks' gestation, Rozé et al. [5] investigated the associations between neonatal intensive care unit (NICU) policies, gut microbiota, and outcomes at 2 years of age. In that study, gut microbiota was determined by 16S ribosomal RNA gene sequencing and classified with regard to the most abundant bacteria present in the stool sample. Six clusters were identified (Fig. 1): cluster 1 was driven by *Enterobacter*, cluster 2 by *Clostridium*, cluster 3 by *Escherichia coli*, cluster 4 by *Enterococcus*, cluster 5 by *Staphylococcus*, and a sixth cluster included non-amplifiable samples owing to low bacterial load. Perinatal determinants were indeed associated with microbiota: clusters 4, 5, and 6 were significantly associated with lower gestational age (26.7 ± 1.8 weeks in average) and cluster 3 with higher mean gestational age (29.4 ± 1.6 weeks, $p < 0.001$). Therefore, cluster 3 appears to correspond to more mature microbiota, and thus was chosen as the reference cluster. Birth by cesarean delivery was associated with increased risk of being in clusters 1, 5, and 6. No assisted ventilation on day 1, direct breastfeeding, and skin-to-skin practice were associated with a more mature cluster. Also, late-onset sepsis occurred significantly more often in clusters 4–6 (56.5, 78.5, and 82.1%, respectively) than in clusters 1–3 (37.7, 14.7, and 21.7%, respectively). In addition, in a subset of the study population, looking for the risk of necrotizing enterocolitis [6], microbiota analysis performed in 16 cases and 78 controls showed an association between *Clostridium neonatale* and *Staphylococcus aureus* (OR: 5.5 [95% CI, 1.4, 20.1] and OR: 7.1 [95% CI, 2.0, 25.0], respectively) [6]. Finally, clusters 4, 5, and 6 were significantly associated with 2-year non-optimal outcome defined by death and/or neurodevelopmental delay using a Global Ages and Stages questionnaire score (aOR, 6.1 [95% CI, 1.5–26.0]; aOR, 4.5 [95% CI, 1.0–20.1]; and aOR, 5.4 [95% CI, 1.4–21.6], respectively) [5]. Overall, the EPIFLORE study shows that gut microbiota of very preterm newborns is not dominated by bifidobacteria in early life, but the development is related to infants' maturity. It is associated with perinatal deter-

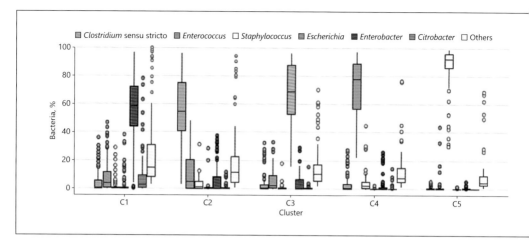

Fig. 1. Gut microbiota grouped into clusters by predominant bacteria in premature infants (5). C1, *Enterobacter* predominant ($n = 240$); C2, *Clostridium* predominant ($n = 68$); C3, *Escherichia* predominant ($n = 61$); C4, *Citrobacter* predominant ($n = 63$); C5, *Staphylococcus* predominant ($n = 52$).

minants, NICU policies such as breastfeeding and skin to skin practice, and may be related to short- and long-term outcome.

Among the factors influencing microbiota, birth mode has been shown to significantly impact microbiota [7]. In a study about maternal secretor genotype of galactoside 2-alpha-L-fucosyltransferase, Korpela et al. [8] showed that a higher level of 2′fucosyllactose (2′FL) in the milk of 76 secretor mothers as compared to 15 non-secretor mothers, may alleviate the effects of caesarian birth on term-infant gut microbiota [8].

In a randomized double-blinded controlled trial, 63 healthy infants received infant formula (control) and were compared to 58 infants fed the same formula with added two human milk oligosaccharides (HMOs), 2′FL and lacto-N-neo-tetraose (LNnT) (test group). Thirty-five breastfed infants served as a reference group [9]. At 3 months of age, microbiota composition in the test group appeared closer to that of breastfed neonates, and the infants were significantly less likely to require antibiotics within their first year of age [9]. In a study of 500 samples of milk from 25 mothers breastfeeding very preterm infants (<32 weeks of gestational age, <1,500 g of birth weight) and 28 mothers breastfeeding term infants, Austin et al. [10] showed that at equivalent postmenstrual age, the concentrations of a number of HMOs, such as 2′FL, were significantly lower in preterm compared to term milk. Finally, in their observational cohort, Gabrielli et al. [11] followed 63 mothers who delivered preterm infants and showed that both 2′FL and LNnT tended to drop through the first month of lactation: com-

Hascoët/Chen

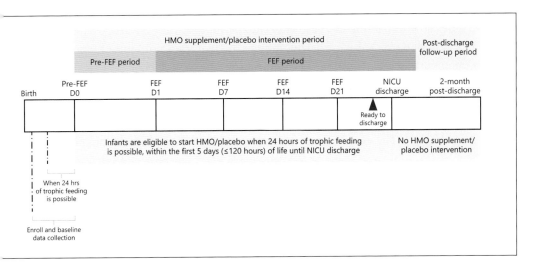

Fig. 2. Intervention study protocol.

pared to preterm colostrum, preterm mature milk generally contained less HMOs, and 2′FL levels were significantly different between values found on day 4 (concentration ranging from 7.23 to 7.36 g/L) and day 30 (concentration ranging from 4.41 to 5.85 g/L, $p < 0.01$).

In summary, prematurity may have a negative impact on gut microbiota and immune and gut functions. HMOs have important physiologic functions in early newborn development. Data support the potential benefit of HMOs in modulating microbiota and suggest that HMOs may alleviate microbiota dysbiosis and reduce the risk of late-onset sepsis and necrotizing enterocolitis in premature infants. Also, prematurity might be associated with lower levels of HMOs in breastmilk. The question then arises of the benefit of HMO supplementation for microbiota and beyond in very premature infants.

To address that question, clinical safety and efficacy data are required. Thus, a multicenter randomized controlled intervention study of the effect of a liquid supplement containing 2 HMOs (2′FL and LNnT) in preterm infants, 27–33 weeks' gestation with a birth weight below 1,700 g, was set up. Proposed HMO dosage distribution (2′FL: LNnT = 10:1) is reflective of the relative amounts found in preterm and term breast milk.

The primary objective of the study is to demonstrate feeding tolerance among preterm infants measured by non-inferiority in days to reach full enteral feeding (FEF) in the HMO versus the placebo group. Shorter time to reach FEF would be an indication of adequate gastro-intestinal tolerance and help to provide sufficient nutrition to assure growth and impact the outcome. Secondary outcome includes growth parameters, gastrointestinal symptoms, any adverse events up to 12 months corrected age, fecal microbiota, gut maturation/immune biomarker outcome and breastmilk HMO composition.

The study design is a multicenter, prospective, randomized, double-blind, controlled trial in 27–33 weeks' gestation infants. Early administration of the products occurs after 24-h trophic feeding and within the first 5 days of postnatal age (Fig. 2). The experimental group receives liquid supplement containing the 2 HMOs (2′FL and LNnT at 0.34 and 0.034 g/kg/day, respectively) in a colorless and odorless solution of 260 mOsm/kg, in addition to regular feeding. The control group receives liquid placebo containing glucose only (0.14 g/kg/day) matched to the experimental product for energy intake and comparable in color, odor, and viscosity. FEF is defined as both enteral feeding volume of at least 150 mL/kg/day and parenteral nutrition discontinuation.

Forty-three infants were included in each group. Gestational age was (mean ± standard deviation) 29.7 ± 1.4 versus 30.2 ± 1.4 weeks in the experimental versus control group, respectively. Both groups were comparable for weight for age z-score at –0.37 ± 0.72 versus –0.56 ± 0.76, length for age z-score at –0.42 ± 0.98 versus –0.46 ± 0.91 and head circumference for age z-score at –0.44 ± 0.91 versus –0.27 ± 1.14, respectively. There was no difference for the sex ratio (42 vs. 44% female) or cesarian section delivery (65 vs. 58%). Data analysis is ongoing and will evaluate the gastrointestinal tolerance parameters, intake of HMOs from human milk, long-term growth outcomes, fecal microbiota, and fecal biomarkers of gut maturation and immunity such as fecal calprotectin, α-1 antitrypsin, and sIgA, as well as adverse events up until 12 months of corrected age.

In conclusion, in premature infants, gut microbiota may show different patterns related to NICU practices and maturity and may be associated with morbidity and outcome. Microbiota appears to be associated with HMOs in preemies. However, prematurity might be associated with lower level of HMOs in breastmilk and lower intake of human milk in early life. Thus, HMO supplementation, given as soon as possible after birth may help reduce dysbiosis leading to more mature microbiota. An intervention study with ongoing analysis will address that question.

Acknowledgments

We thank Doctors Jean-Marc Jellimann, Marie Chevallier, Catherine Gire, Roselyne Brat, Jean-Christophe Rozé, Karine Norbert, Jelena Buncic-Markovic, Mickaël Hartweg, and Claude Billeaud for their participation in the realization of the intervention trial.

Conflict of Interest Statement

J.M.H. received a honorarium for his participation to the NNI96 Workshop.

References

1   Harmsen HJM, Wildeboer-Veloo ACM, Raangs GC, et al. Analysis of intestinal flora development in breast-fed and formula-fed infants by using molecular identification and detection methods. J Pediatr Gastroenterol Nutr. 2000 Jan;30(1):61–7.

2   Wharton BA, Balmer SE, Scott PH. Sorrento studies of diet and fecal flora in the newborn. Pediatr Int. 1994 Oct;36(5):579–84.

3   Hascoët J-M, Hubert C, Rochat F, et al. Effect of formula composition on the development of infant gut microbiota. J Pediatr Gastroenterol Nutr. 2011 Jun;52(6):756–62.

4   Newburg DS, He Y. Neonatal gut microbiota and human milk glycans cooperate to attenuate infection and inflammation. Clin Obstet Gynecol. 2015 Dec;58(4):814–26.

5   Rozé JC, Ancel PY, Marchand-Martin L, et al. Assessment of neonatal intensive care unit practices and preterm newborn gut microbiota and 2-year neurodevelopmental outcomes. JAMA Netw Open. 2020 Sep;3(9):e2018119.

6   Rozé JC, Ancel PY, Lepage P, et al. Nutritional strategies and gut microbiota composition as risk factors for necrotizing enterocolitis in very-preterm infants. Am J Clin Nutr. 2017;106(3):821–30.

7   Bäckhed F, Roswall J, Peng Y, et al. Dynamics and stabilization of the human gut microbiome during the first year of life. Cell Host Microbe. 2015 Jun;17(6):852.

8   Korpela K, Salonen A, Hickman B, et al. Fucosylated oligosaccharides in mother's milk alleviate the effects of caesarean birth on infant gut microbiota. Sci Rep. 2018 Dec;8(1):13757.

9   Berger B, Porta N, Foata F, et al. Linking human milk oligosaccharides, infant fecal community types, and later risk to require antibiotics. mBio. 2020 Mar;11(2):e03196–19.

10 Austin S, De Castro CA, Sprenger N, et al. Human milk oligosaccharides in the milk of mothers delivering term versus preterm infants. Nutrients. 2019 Jun;11(6):1282.

11 Gabrielli O, Zampini L, Galeazzi T, et al. Preterm milk oligosaccharides during the first month of lactation. Pediatrics. 2011 Dec;128(6):e1520–31.

Jean-Michel Hascoët
Service de Néonatologie
Maternité Régionale Universitaire A. Pinard
10 rue du Dr Heydenreich
FR -54035 Nancy
France
jean-michel.hascoet@univ-lorraine.fr

Published online: May 10, 2022

Embleton ND, Haschke F, Bode L (eds): Strategies in Neonatal Care to Promote Optimized Growth and Development: Focus on Low Birth Weight Infants. 96th Nestlé Nutrition Institute Workshop, May 2021. Nestlé Nutr Inst Workshop Ser. Basel, Karger, 2022, vol 96, pp 166–174 (DOI: 10.1159/000519401)

Human Milk Bioactives: Future Perspective

Kristen L. Finn[a]   Brian D. Kineman[a]   Laura A. Czerkies[a]
Ryan S. Carvalho[b]

[a]Gerber, Nestlé Nutrition, Arlington, VA, USA; [b]Nestlé Nutrition, Vevey, Switzerland

Abstract

Human milk is a dynamic, complex fluid that offers much more than nutrition to infants. The macronutrient content of human milk has been well characterized and described. However, human milk is not a simple matrix of protein, carbohydrate, fat, and micronutrients. The National Institutes of Health have defined bioactives in food as elements that "affect biological processes or substrates and hence have an impact on body function or condition and ultimately health." Bioactives are cells, anti-infectious and anti-inflammatory agents, growth factors, and prebiotics that are naturally present in human milk. They may explain the differences in health outcomes observed between breastfed and non-breastfed infants. They influence the development of the immune and gastrointestinal systems, gut microbiota, neurodevelopment, metabolic health, and protection against infection. Human milk oligosaccharides are one bioactive that have been an increasingly popular area of research. This review provides a broad overview of some bioactive components that positively affect the immune system and touches on certain well-known growth factors present in human milk. Future research will look at the interplay of the multitude of bioactive components in human milk as a biological system and beyond singular compounds.

© 2022 S. Karger AG, Basel

Introduction

Human milk is a complex, dynamic fluid providing ideal nutrition for the human infant and is uniquely designed for each mother-infant dyad. Beyond providing majority of macronutrients and micronutrients at optimal levels for growth and development, it is a source of nutrition containing bioactive components that serve a variety of biological functions, including development of the immune and gastrointestinal systems, gut microbiota, neurodevelopment, metabolic health, and protection against infection. The bioactive cells, anti-infectious and anti-inflammatory agents, growth factors, and prebiotics that are naturally present in human milk may explain the differences in health outcomes observed between breastfed and non-breastfed infants throughout the ages.

Nutritive Components of Human Milk

The composition of human milk changes throughout lactation stages from colostrum to late lactation, varying within feeds and between mothers. Despite variations in maternal nutrition, macronutrient composition of human milk is remarkably conserved across populations with the mean macronutrient composition of mature, term milk estimated to be approximately 0.9–1.2 g/dL for protein, 3.2–3.6 g/dL for fat, and 6.7–7.8 g/dL for lactose. Energy estimates range from 65 to 70 kcal/dL [1]. Lactose is the primary carbohydrate source of human milk, and the carbohydrate content of human milk is the least variable of the macronutrients. Human milk fat is more variable in human milk, even within a feed, where the fat content of hindmilk (milk expressed at the end of a feed) can be two to three times greater than that of foremilk (milk expressed at the beginning of a feed). Palmitic and oleic acids are the dominant fatty acids in human milk. The fatty acid profile of human milk varies in relation to maternal diet, particularly in the long-chain polyunsaturated fatty acids. Casein and whey are the main protein components of human milk, and the ratio of these two changes over the course of lactation where human milk is predominantly whey in early lactation and closer to a 50:50 whey:casein ratio in late lactation. Protein levels decrease over time in human milk and are less affected by maternal diet. Micronutrient content of human milk can be dependent on maternal diet and stores, including vitamins A, B_1, B_2, B_6, B_{12}, D, and iodine. As the maternal diet may not always be optimal, use of a multivitamin during lactation is often recommended. Even with supplementation, vitamins K and D are often present at low levels in human milk, and therefore a vitamin K injection at birth is recommended by the American Academy of Pediatrics as well as supplementation of vitamin D in the breastfed infant [1].

Bioactive Components of Human Milk

Bioactive components of food have been defined as elements that "affect biological processes or substrates and hence have an impact on body function or condition and ultimately health" [2]. As defined by the NIH, bioactive food components are constituents in foods or dietary supplements, other than those needed to meet basic human nutritional needs, that are responsible for changes in health status [3]. The commonality of these definitions is that the focus is on the impact on health, not on the nutritive aspect of the food component, such as providing energy or protein.

Human milk has thousands of bioactive components coming from a variety of sources. Some are secreted by the mammary epithelium, some are produced by cells present in the milk, and others are transported across the mammary epithelium from maternal serum [1]. Milk fat globule that is present in human milk and secreted by the mammary epithelium also contains membrane-bound proteins and lipids that it brings into human milk [4].

Broad categories of bioactive components in breastmilk include immunological and growth factors. Immunological factors include immune cells such as T cells and lymphocytes, cytokines, secretory immunoglobulin A (sIgA), and human milk oligosaccharides (HMOs) [1]. Growth factors include growth- and metabolism-regulating hormones like calcitonin and adiponectin in addition to bioactive proteins such as insulin like growth factor, vascular endothelial growth factor, and neuronal growth factors [1].

Human Milk Oligosaccharides

HMOs represent a vast, functional component of human milk making up the third most abundant proportion of the solid components of milk surpassed in concentration only by lactose and lipids. The oligosaccharide content of human milk varies between 10–15 g per liter (g/L) of mature milk and 20–25 g/L of colostrum [5, 6]. They are predominantly present in free form in human milk and in this free form are customarily called HMOs. Although some of these structures are also present in the milk of other mammals, oligosaccharides are much more abundant in human milk [5].

HMOs are comprised of a linear or branched elongation of lactose by the building blocks fucose, sialic acid, and N-acetylglucosamine. HMOs are generally classified into four different categories: non-fucosylated, non-sialylated (neutral), fucosylated, non-sialylated (fucosylated, neutral), non-fucosylated, sialylated (acidic), fucosylated, sialylated (fucosylated acidic) [5]. Over 150 unique structures have been analytically separated, but about 20 structures comprise the major portion of HMOs with the remaining glycans representing a smaller fraction [5, 7]. Individual variation of milk oligosaccharides can partially be explained by material genetics, and this is well characterized by expression of two fucosyltransferases: FUT2 (secreter gene) and FUT3 (Lewis gene) [5]. Both are polymorphic with different alleles being responsible for the non-secretor (FUT2–/–) and Lewis negative (FUT3–/–) types. Milk of secretor women is abundant in 2′-fucosyllactose (2′FL), LNFP I, and other α1–2-fucosylated HMOs. In contrast, non-secretors lack the functional FUT2 enzyme, and their milk contains very little α1–2-fucosylated HMOs but does contain other fucosylated HMOs [8]. HMO content may also be influenced by nongenetic maternal and infant factors. Lactation stage, maternal BMI, maternal age, maternal diet, mode of delivery, parity, infant gestational age, and infant sex have all been suggested as factors that determine individual variation in milk oligosaccharide content [9].

A number of biological and physiological benefits have been attributed to HMOs, and these roles are mainly characterized on the basis of protective properties that comprise an innate defense system for infants [5]. HMOs are selective substrates for specific intestinal bacteria, protect against infection by blocking pathogen attachment to epithelial cells, promote immunomodulatory activity, and improve gut barrier function [10].

The majority of ingested HMOs reach the large intestine where they provide selective substrates for specific gut bacteria. This prebiotic activity of HMOs is best characterized among specific bifidobacteria species, which have the capability to transport them for internal digestion or secrete glycosidases that externally hydrolyze HMOs to byproduct constituents that can be metabolized by the bacterium [11]. *Bifidobacterium longum* subsp *infantis* has a gene that expresses not only glycosidases, but also sugar transporters and glycan-binding proteins likely linked to HMO metabolism [11]. *B. breve*, or *B. bifidum* strains have also been shown to grow in the presence of select HMOs [12, 13]. HMOs metabolize into short-chain fatty acids including butyrate, the preferred energy source for colon epithelial cells, contributing to the maintenance of the gut barrier [14].

HMOs can also inhibit pathogens by competitive binding with the host cell surface receptor [15]. HMOs have been shown to provide protection against a wide spectrum of pathogens, including those associated with diarrheal, respiratory, and urinary infections and human immunodeficiency virus [16].

An increasing number of in vitro studies suggest that HMOs also exert effects independent of microbiota, by directly modulating immune responses by affecting immune cell populations and cytokine secretion [10]. HMOs may either act locally on cells of the mucosa-associated lymphoid tissues or on a systemic level [5]. When cord blood T cells are exposed to sialylated HMOs, the resulting lymphocyte response was suggestive of lymphocyte maturation and a shift toward a more balanced Th1/Th2 cytokine production [17]. In regard to neutral oligosaccharides, significant associations between levels of 2'FL in mothers' breast milk and "any allergic disease," IgE-associated disease, eczema, and IgE-associated eczema in C-section-born infants have been reported [18].

HMOs have been considered as potentially important components in support of brain development and cognitive function. The predominance of the research in this area has focused on the role of sialylated HMOs, an important source of sialic acid in infancy [19]. However, 2'FL may specifically have an important role in early cognitive development. Vazquez et al. [20] studied the ability of 2'FL, specifically, to affect learning in a small trial of mice and rats evaluating excitatory postsynaptic potentials, various types of learning, and behavior. The results demonstrated that dietary 2'-FL exerts a positive effect on learning and memory in rodents [21, 22].

Immunological Function of Bioactives in Human Milk
The level of immunological components of breastmilk varies in the first year of life. For example, α-lactalbumin declines gradually over time with significantly lower levels in mature milk at 4–8 months of life compared to the first few days of life. Other immune factors such as lactoferrin, immunoglobulins, and transforming growth factor β1 (TGF-β1) follow a similar pattern with significantly higher levels in very early milk compared to mature milk at 2–4 weeks of life, and then remain relatively stable over the first year of life. TGF-β2 follows a slightly different pattern, declining significantly over the first month of life but then fluctuating throughout the first year [23]. The high levels of immunological components and relatively low levels of lactose and some micronutrients in colostrum suggest that its evolutionary function is more immunological than nutritive [1].

Human milk contains many immune cells such as T cells, stem cells, lymphocytes, and macrophages that originate from the mother's mature immune system, migrating from the bloodstream to the mammary epithelium. Although the quantity of these cells differs between individuals, infants consume roughly ten billion immune cells daily in early lactation; roughly 80% of which are macrophages [1]. In addition to pathogen phagocytosis, breastmilk macrophages have unique functions including the ability to convert into dendritic cells which then stimulate the infant's immune system via T-cell activity [1, 24]. About 6% of cells in human milk are stem cells which can differentiate into multiple tissue types and may be involved in the development of the infant's immune cells [25]. During infection of either the mother or infant, an increase in leukocytes has been observed indicating a protective function of leukocytes for the infant [24].

Immunoglobulins are central to the passive transfer of immunity from mother to infant [26]. sIgA is the most abundant immunoglobulin in human milk making up over 90% of total immunoglobulins, although levels decline over time

[24, 27]. Other immunoglobulins, such as immunoglobulin M follows a similar pattern whereas immunoglobulin G is higher in mature milk compared to transitional milk [27]. Maternal sIgA provides passive immunity by binding to pathogens and blocking infection as well as facilitating their removal by entrapping them in mucus [24]. Not only does maternal sIgA provide passive immunity, it stimulates the infant immune system via dendritic cell activation without stimulating an inflammatory response [1, 28].

Human milk is the primary source of lactoferrin in the infant gut [29]. It is known for having antibacterial, antimicrobial, antiviral, antiparasitic, antifungal, antioxidant, anti-inflammatory, and even anticancerous properties [29]. Since a major role of lactoferrin is to transport iron in the plasma, it has a strong iron binding capability enabling it to withhold iron from iron dependent pathogens [29, 30]. Lactoferrin receptors on the mucosal surface of intestinal cells allow for lactoferrin to enter the intestinal microvilli where it stimulates the immune response by inducing leukocyte activity such as increased natural killer cell and phagocyte activity. Lactoferrin has also been shown to increase and decrease production of proinflammatory cytokines, dendritic cells, T cells, and B cells [29].

Osteopontin is present in most human tissues and fluids but is most abundant in human milk. Osteopontin is involved in several biological functions including bone remodeling, inhibiting calcification of soft tissues, and plays an important role in the development of immune response and modulation. It has been hypothesized that osteopontin attaches to monocytes directing them to sites acting as a transporter. It influences the function of other immune cells such as macrophages, T cells, and dendritic cells. It also has antibacterial properties, binding itself to foreign microorganisms making them more susceptible to phagocytosis [31].

Gangliosides are present in almost all human tissues and play a pivotal role in infant growth and immune response. Total ganglioside concentration is significantly higher in mature milk compared to colostrum but is highly variable between individuals. Gangliosides follow different trajectories over time with GD2 decreasing and GM3 increasing over the course of lactation [32]. They act as decoy receptors for pathogens preventing binding to intestinal cells. They also play a role in immune system development such as influencing the production of IgA and cytokines as well as promoting maturation of dendritic cells [33].

Reactive oxygen species (ROS) are molecules that participate in cellular signaling pathways, but in excess can cause cellular damage. To combat this, the body has a variety of antioxidant systems to maintain the balance between ROS and antioxidants. If excessive ROS production occurs or insufficient antioxidant systems persist, the result is oxidative stress. Examples of endogenous antioxidants are enzymatic proteins like superoxide dismutase or glutathione peroxidase. Other examples are those antioxidants found in foods such as vitamins and carotenoids. All these examples plus more are present in human milk to help the infant combat excessive ROS and protect against disease. Levels of antioxidants range, depending on time of collection and geographic site of collection. The total antioxidant capacity of human milk seems to be higher in colostrum compared to mature milk [25].

Bioactives Affecting Growth

In addition to the immunological impact human milk bioactives impart on the infant, human milk contains a variety of growth factors. Growth factors such as epidermal growth factor, growth hormone and insulin-like growth factor-1 are present in human milk and affect the morphology and function of the gastrointestinal tract [34, 35]. Insulin-like growth factor 1 and its binding proteins also play a role in programming infant growth trajectories due to their well-established roles in linear growth, and body composition [36]. Brain-derived neurotrophic factor and glial cell-line derived neurotrophic factor are neuronal growth factors found in human milk that play a role in the maturation of the enteric nervous system [37]. Adipokines are cytokines from adipocytes that modify weight gain and body composition in infants that have long-term effects on metabolic programming and are involved in regulation of food intake and energy balance. Examples include adiponectin, ghrelin, and leptin. Adiponectin tends to be the most abundant and is a multifunctional hormone that regulates metabolism and suppresses inflammation. Human milk adiponectin also seems to have an influence on infant growth [25]. Human milk contains many other growth factors beyond those mentioned here affecting the vascular, neuronal, and other organ systems of the infant [1].

Factors That Influence Bioactives in Human Milk

There are several maternal factors that influence the quantity, quality, and composition of bioactives in human milk. These would include physical factors such as genotype, body mass index, physiologic state, and underlying medical conditions, environmental factors such diet, mode of delivery, medication use, and other factors such as infant gestational age and stage of lactation [9, 38]. Influencing modifiable factors may optimize human milk such that it improves infant outcomes ranging from infectious and allergic diseases to cognitive, gastrointestinal, and immune system development.

Conclusions

The evolving research surrounding bioactives in human milk offers much promise in our understanding of the many and unique benefits of breastfeeding. While this review described some of the individual bioactive components of human milk, a more comprehensive view of human milk as a biological system is needed as each component likely does not act independently. Future research is needed focusing on the inter-relation and complex relations between bioactive components. The next generation of research should also focus on how modifiable maternal factors influence human milk bioactive composition. Finally, research is needed on the role of bioactives in the health and development of high-risk populations such as preterm and medically fragile infants. Major strides are being undertaken to explore and increase the research being conducted to gain a better understanding of human milk and its complexities and fluidity to optimally nourish infants [39].

Conflict of Interest Statement

K.L.F., B.D.K., L.A.C. and R.S.C. are employees of Nestlé Nutrition.

References

1 Ballard O, Morrow AL. Human milk composition: nutrition and bioactive factors. Pediatr Clin North Am. 2013;60(1):49–74.
2 Schrezenmeir J, Korhonen H, Williams C, et al. Foreword. Br J Nutr. 2000;84(1):S1.
3 NIH, Office of Dietary Supplements. Federal Register Vol. 69 No. 179 FR Dec 04-20892, Sept 16, 2004 [cited 2021 Sept 6]. Available from: ods.od.nih/gov/Research/Bioactive_Food_Components_Initiative.aspx.
4 Cavaletto M, Giuffrida MG, Conti A. The proteomic approach to analysis of human fat globule membrane. Clin Chim Acta. 2004;347(1–2):41–8.
5 Bode L. Human milk oligosaccharides: every baby needs a sugar mama. Glycobiology. 2012;22:1147–62.
6 Kunz C, Kuntz S, Rudloff S. Bioactivity of human milk oligosaccharides. In: Moreno FM, Sanz ML, editors. Food Oligosaccharides: Production, Analysis and Bioactivity. Chichester: John Wiley & Sons; 2014. pp 5–20.
7 Thurl S, Munzert M, Henker J, et al. Variation of human milk oligosaccharides in relation to milk groups and lactational periods. Br J Nutr. 2010;104:1261–71.
8 Thurl S, Henker J, Siegel M, et al. Detection of four human milk groups with respect to Lewis blood group dependent oligosaccharides. Glycoconj J. 1997;14:795–9.
9 Han SM, Derraik J, Binia A, et al. Maternal and infant factors influencing human milk oligosaccharide composition: beyond maternal genetics. J Nutr. 2021;151(6):1383–93.
10 Donovan SM, Comstock SS. Human milk oligosaccharides influence neonatal mucosal and systemic immunity. Ann Nutr Metab. 2016;69(Suppl 2):42–51.
11 Milani C, Duranti S, Bottacini F, et al. The first microbial colonizers of the human gut: composition, activities, and health implications of the infant gut microbiota. Microbiol Mol Biol Rev. 2017;81(4):e00036–17.
12 Marcobal A, Barboza M, Froehlich JW, et al. Consumption of human milk oligosaccharides by gut-related microbes. J Agric Food Chem. 2010;58:5334–40.

13 Asakuma S, Hatakeyama E, Urashima T, et al. Physiology of consumption of human milk oligosaccharides by infant gut-associated bifidobacteria. J Biol Chem. 2011;286:34583–92.

14 Rivière A, Selak M, Lantin D, et al. Bifidobacteria and butyrate-producing colon bacteria: importance and strategies for their stimulation in the human gut. Front Microbiol. 2016;7:979.

15 Newburg DS. Oligosaccharides in human milk and bacterial colonization. J Pediatr Gastroenterol Nutr. 2000;30(Suppl 2):S8–S17.

16 Asadpoor M, Peeters C, Henricks PA, et al. Antipathogenic functions of non-digestible oligosaccharides in vitro. Nutrients. 2020;12(6):1789.

17 Eiwegger T, Stahl B, Schmitt J, et al. Human milk-derived oligosaccharides and plant-derived oligosaccharides stimulate cytokine production of cord blood T-cells in vitro. Pediatr Res. 2004;56:536–40.

18 Sprenger N, Odenwald H, Kukkonen AK, et al. FUT2-dependent breast milk oligosaccharides and allergy at 2 and 5 years of age in infants with high hereditary allergy risk. Eur J Nutr. 2017;56:1293–301.

19 ten Bruggencate SJ, Bovee-Oudenhoven IM, Feitsma AL, et al. Functional role and mechanisms of sialyllactose and other sialylated milk oligosaccharides. Nutr Rev. 2014;72:377–89.

20 Vázquez E, Barranco A, Ramírez M, et al. Effects of a human milk oligosaccharide, 2'-fucosyllactose, on hippocampal long-term potentiation and learning capabilities in rodents. J Nutr Biochem. 2015;26(5):455–65.

21 Berger PK, Plows JF, Jones RB, et al. Human milk oligosaccharide 2′-fucosyllactose links feedings at 1 month to cognitive development at 24 months in infants of normal and overweight mothers. PLoS One. 2020;15(2):e0228323.

22 Oliveros E, Martín MJ, Torres-Espínola FJ, et al. Human milk levels of 2′-fucosyllactose and 6′-sialyllactose are positively associated with infant neurodevelopment and are not impacted by maternal BMI or diabetic status. J Nutr Food Sci. 2021;4:024.

23 Affolter M, Garcia-Rodenas CL, Vinyes-Pares G, et al. Temporal changes of protein composition in breast milk of Chinese urban mothers and impact of caesarean section delivery. Nutrients. 2016;8:504.

24 Cacho NT, Lawrence RM. Innate immunity and breast milk. Front Immunol. 2017;8:584.

25 Gila-Diaz A, Arribas SM, Algara A, et al. A review of bioactive factors in human breastmilk: a focus on prematurity. Nutrients. 2019;11:1307.

26 Hurley WL, Theil PK. Perspectives on immunoglobulins in colostrum and milk. Nutrients. 2011;3(4):442–74.

27 Gao X, McMahon RJ, Woo JG, et al. Temporal changes in milk proteomes reveal developing milk functions. J Proteome Res. 2012;11(7):3897–907.

28 Kadaoui KA, Corthésy. Secretory IgA mediates bacterial translocation to dendritic cells in mouse Peyer's patches with restriction to mucosal compartment. J Immunol. 2007;179(11):7751–7.

29 Kanwar JR, Roy K, Patel Y, et al. Multifunctional iron bound lactoferrin and nanomedicinal approaches to enhance its bioactive functions. Molecules. 2015;20:9703–31.

30 Lonnerdal B. Bioactive proteins in human milk: health, nutrition, and implications for infant formulas. J Pediatr. 2016;173S:S4–S9.

31 Schack L, Lange A, Kelsen J, et al. Considerable variation in the concentration of osteopontin in human milk, bovine milk, and infant formulas. J Diet Sci. 2009;92(11):578–85.

32 Giuffrida F, Cruz-Hernandez C, Bertschy E, et al. Temporal changes of human breast milk lipids of Chinese mothers. Nutrients. 2016;8:17.

33 Rueda R. The role of dietary gangliosides on immunity and the prevention of infection. Br J Nutr. 2007;98(Suppl 1):S68–S73.

34 Hirai C, Ichiba H, Saito M, et al. Trophic effect of multiple growth factors in amniotic fluid or human milk on cultured human fetal small intestinal cells. J Pediatr Gastroenterol Nutr. 2002;34(5):524–8.

35 Dvorak B. Milk epidermal growth factor and gut protection. J Pediatr. 2010;156(2 Suppl):S31–S35.

36 Hoeflich A, Meyer Z. Functional analysis of the IGF-system in milk. Best Pract Res Clin Endocrinol Metab. 2017(31):409–18.

37 Rodrigues D, Li A, Nair D, Blennerhassett M. Glial cell line-derived neurotrophic factor is a key neurotrophin in the postnatal enteric nervous system. Neurogastroenterol Motil. 2011;23:e44–e56.

38 Samuel TM, Zhou Q, Giuffrida F, et al. Nutritional and non-nutritional composition of human milk is modulated by maternal, infant, and methodological factors. Front Nutr. 2020;7:576133.

39 Christian P, Smith ER, Lee SE, et al. The need to study human milk as a biological system. Am J Clin Nutr. 2021;113:1063–1072.

Ryan S. Carvalho
Nestlé Nutrition
Avenue Nestle 55
CH–1800 Vevey
Switzerland
ryan.carvalho@nestle.com

Published online: May 10, 2022

Embleton ND, Haschke F, Bode L (eds): Strategies in Neonatal Care to Promote Optimized Growth and Development: Focus on Low Birth Weight Infants. 96th Nestlé Nutrition Institute Workshop, May 2021. Nestlé Nutr Inst Workshop Ser. Basel, Karger, 2022, vol 96, pp 175–177 (DOI: 10.1159/000519405)

Summary on the Role of Human Milk Oligosaccharides and the Microbiome in the Health of Very Low Birth Weight Infants

The health of very low birth weight infants is often challenged by immature tissues and organ systems including the gut and immune system paired with an unusual environment of a premature extrauterine life. Preterm birth comes with premature exposure to microbes that start to colonize the infant gut and other niches early and under "unnatural" conditions. A healthy colonization is important both for the immediate as well as the long-term health and development of the host. An unhealthy colonization or dysbiosis can lead to severe immediate complications like necrotizing enterocolitis (NEC) and have long-lasting consequences with increased risk of obesity, allergy, asthma, and other disorders later in life. Therefore, developing healthy host-microbe interactions early in life represents a major challenge for infant health in general and the health of very low birth weight infants in particular. At the same time, challenges create opportunities for potential interventions to help shape healthy microbial communities. Interventions include the use of human milk, the use of specific human milk bioactives like human milk oligosaccharides (HMOs), as well as the use of probiotics and synbiotics.

Human milk feeding is often the primary driver of shaping microbial communities early in life. Within human milk, HMOs represent the third most abundant components after lactose and lipids. These complex carbohydrates serve as prebiotics and as such provide select bacteria with metabolic substrates to thrive, while other bacteria are less likely to grow because they cannot utilize this abundant carbohydrate source. Among the bacteria that can utilize some or all HMOs are some Bifidobacteria strains as well as some Bacteroides strains, and both have been associated with improved infant health and, as a consequence, are under investigation as suitable probiotic interventions.

However, HMOs are more than just "food for bugs." In addition, HMOs have antimicrobial effects on potential pathogens, but also directly modulate epithelial and immune cell responses independent of microbes. For example, several independent cohort studies on mothers and preterm infants have shown that the HMO disialyllacto-N-tetraose (DSLNT) is significantly associated with decreased NEC risk. While mere associations in cohort studies do not prove causality, results from NEC animal models with HMO interventions corroborate the findings that DSLNT protects against NEC. The effects are highly structure-specific with HMOs other than DSLNT being ineffective in the animal model and also not showing positive associations in any of the human cohort studies. This high structure-specificity points to a direct, receptor-mediated effect on host or microbial cells and raises three major questions: (i) How do we translate HMO interventions for term and preterm infants to clinical applications? (ii) Can we develop targeted synbiotics that contain beneficial probiotics that thrive on some but not all HMOs and leave other HMOs like DSLNT intact so they can exert their microbe-independent functions? (iii) Can we leverage bioactive components other than HMOs to improve the health of very low birth weight infants.

The first chapter in this third session introduces the interplay of HMOs with microbes and highlights the importance of host-microbe interactions and the gut microbiome for immediate and long-term health with a particular focus on very low birth infants, NEC, and sepsis. The chapter also introduces novel in vitro and ex vivo organoid systems that allow researchers to take a closer look at host-microbe interactions on a molecular and cellular level and how we can interfere with milk bioactives.

Most HMOs are uniquely present in human milk and are not found in the milk of other mammals or anywhere else in nature. However, recent advances in biotechnology enabled the production of select HMOs at large scale and fairly low cost. The second chapter summarizes the design and results from randomized controlled trials with specific HMOs like 2′fucosyllactose and/or lacto-N-neotetraose added to infant formulas for term infants.

While several studies with HMO supplementation in healthy term infants have been completed, infant immaturity, milk composition, and environment are very different for very low birth weight infants, and so is their microbiome. The third chapter summarizes what we know about the gut microbiome in very low birth weight infants and outlines an ongoing multicenter randomized controlled intervention study with a supplement containing two HMOs that evaluates gastrointestinal tolerance, long-term growth, effects on fecal microbiota composition as well as gut maturation and immunity.

Last but not least, human milk is more than just HMOs. Although oligosaccharides are a major component that is under intense investigation, human milk contains many other bioactive molecules that are introduced in the fourth and last chapter of this session. While many of these human milk bioactives alone can have a beneficial effect, it is important to emphasize that none of these components occur and act in isolation, they interact with other milk components in a complex system. In fact, human milk itself does also not stand in isolation and is part of a dynamic biological system consistent of the mother-milk-infant triad which is embedded in socioeconomic, cultural, behavioral, and environmental contexts. And once again, both the triad as well as the contexts are very different in healthy term infants compared to very low birth weight infants. Future research needs to acknowledge that individual milk components and human milk itself cannot be studied in isolation but need to be thoroughly investigated as part of a biological system in a specific context. Only then will we be able to fully leverage human milk bioactives such as HMOs as well as probiotics and targeted synbiotics to improve the health of very low birth weight infants.

Lars Bode

Subject Index

Insulin-like growth factor-1 (IGF-1)
    amino acids in secretion 90
    brain development role 26
    milk 172
    retinopathy of prematurity protection 29
Intraventricular hemorrhage (IVH), docosahexaenoic acid supplementation
    outcomes 113
Iron, supplementation in preterm infants 131–133
IVH, *see* Intraventricular hemorrhage

Lactoferrin, milk immune function 171
Late-onset sepsis (LOS)
    docosahexaenoic acid supplementation outcomes 113
    enteral feeding outcomes in preterm infants 2, 4–6
    microbial dysfunction 143
LOS, *see* Late-onset sepsis

Magnetic resonance imaging (MRI), body composition assessment in infants 46, 47
Metabolic syndrome, risk from preterm birth 50
Microbiota, *see* Gut microbiome
Milk tolerance, enteral feeding guidance
    blood transfusion 7
    feed intolerance 8
    infant factors 7
    patent ductus arteriosus 7, 8
MOBYDIck trial 110, 111, 113
Mother's own milk, *see* Breast milk
MRI, *see* Magnetic resonance imaging

NEC, *see* Necrotizing enterocolitis
Necrotizing enterocolitis (NEC)
    body composition effects 50
    donor milk and outcomes 68
    enteral feeding outcomes in preterm infants 2, 4–6
    human milk and probiotic studies 144, 145, 176
    microbial dysfunction 143, 175
    neurocognitive outcomes 28, 66
Neurodevelopment, *see* Cognition

Osteopenia, preterm infants 133, 134
Osteopontin, milk immune function 171
Oxidative stress
    early-life stress 121
    milk antioxidants 171, 172

Parenteral nutrition, PEPaNIC trial 20
Pasteurization, *see* Donor milk
Patent ductus arteriosus (PDA), enteral feeding considerations 7, 8